PRAISE FOR *The Addict*

"A gripping, illuminating book. . . . Dr. Stein is drawn, in an almost Sherlock Holmesian way, toward trying to fathom and analyze addicts' behavior. . . . A compelling book. . . . Hauntingly and successfully, Stein lets readers make a doctor's experiences their own."

—Janet Maslin, *New York Times*

"An uncommonly caring doctor points a new way out of addiction. . . . A useful, sensible, and often inspiring guide to how the medical profession does—and should—treat the sick, and the sick at heart."

—Francine Prose, *O, The Oprah Magazine*

"*The Addict* is a beautifully told story of addiction, but from the perspective of a physician whose vast experience working with people caught up in substance abuse reveals itself not in cynicism but in great insight, empathy, and compassion. Stein's experience and his writing skills provide a window to what it is about being human that drives us to addiction and what it takes to be rescued."

—Abraham Verghese, author of
The Tennis Partner, My Own Country,
and *Cutting for Stone*

"The rewarding story of Stein's work to help get one patient on the road to recovery. . . . Vivid. . . . A touching, honest account of one woman's fight with addiction."

—*Boston Globe*

"An eye-opening look into the murky world of addiction."

—*St. Petersburg Times*

"With a crisp detachment that belies his vulnerability and caring, Stein masterfully records the relentless pain—physical and psychological—that brings Lucy Fields, a twenty-nine-year-old Vicodin addict, to his door with 'a peculiarly common modern American condition.' . . . It's Lucy's arc of illness that keeps this haunting narrative moving forward, but it's Stein's clear-eyed compassion that catapults her story from pathetic to sympathetic."

—*Publishers Weekly* (starred review)

PRAISE FOR *The Lonely Patient*

THE
ADDICT

THE
ADDICT

ONE PATIENT, ONE DOCTOR, ONE YEAR

MICHAEL
STEIN

HARPER PERENNIAL

NEW YORK • LONDON • TORONTO • SYDNEY • NEW DELHI • AUCKLAND

HARPER ● PERENNIAL

A hardcover edition of this book was pubished in 2009 by William Morrow, an imprint of HarperCollins Publishers.

HarperCollins books may be purchased for educational, business, or sales promotional use. For information please write: Special Markets Department, HarperCollins Publishers, 10 East 53rd Street, New York, NY 10022.

FIRST HARPER PERENNIAL EDITION PUBLISHED 2010.

Designed by Chris Welch

Library of Congress Cataloging-in-Publication Data has been applied for.

ISBN 978-0-06-136814-1 (pbk.)

10 11 12 13 14   OV/RRD   10 9 8 7 6 5 4 3 2

FOR MY NEPHEWS AND NIECES,

ANNA, SAM, DAVID, ADAM, BEN, IAN, SAM T., AND RACHEL

OFF TO WAR AND AT HOME

People make momentous shifts, but not the changes they imagine.

—*Alice Munro,* Differently

Contents

CONTENTS

PART THREE

Author's Note

As an author of nonfiction who is also a doctor writing about his patients, I have particular storytelling challenges. When I began *The Addict*, I knew I wanted to portray a patient of mine, a young woman whose story touched me deeply. I knew that I would have to change names, places, and many details of her life to protect her privacy. If she were ever to read this book, I wanted her to remember things about herself but feel safely disguised. My goal was to illuminate her story while widening her view and other readers' views of addiction.

I am not a journalist; I am a doctor. As a writer, I have a very different relationship with my subjects than a journalist might, because what I learn from patients is personal and medical, and it is not solicited with publication in mind. I never audiotape my interviews, but I occasionally take notes.

Beyond the requirements of journalism, but in keeping with my medical oath, I had to guard the confidentiality of all the patients included in these pages. This was of great importance to me and at times it conflicted with my oath as a writer—to give readers the most realistic sense as possible of an addict's psychology and behavior from a doctor's point of view. In writing about the patient whom I discuss most extensively here, I gave her some experiences and characteristics that belong to other patients. The main challenge was to tell true stories that my patients would recognize but not feel betrayed by in their reading.

Just as there is no single right way to help addicts, there is no single perspective that captures the entire feel of addiction. I have tried to illustrate the range and variety of terrible moments and encouraging successes my patients live through. This is the story of one addict, but it is also the story of all addicts.

PART I

CHAPTER 1

Wednesday, April 16

It had rained the first week in April that year, and though the reappearance of the sun raised the temperature to only forty-five New England degrees, it made me hopeful again. My new patient sat on her black Converse high-tops, her legs tucked under, as if she was trying to keep herself from running away. She appeared to be in her late twenties and was wearing a loose gray sweater over a pink and green polka-dot blouse. With her chin tipped into her collar, eyes toward the floor, she appeared shy, or embarrassed. She was tall but slight and had rolled up her sleeves to the elbows.

"I'm here for your program," she said. "You still have openings, right?" Her soft voice gave me an impression of politeness.

Sixty minutes isn't enough time to learn a patient's complicated history so I was happy to start at a gallop. I was grateful she required no transition from the general cheerfulness of just meeting each other to the serious conversation, filled with effort and nervousness and specifics, that would constitute the rest of the hour. The answer to her first question was a simple yes or no.

"Yes, I do," I answered, as if we were getting married, which in some sense, we were; from that moment forward, our time together would, like any pair's, get snagged on expectations, hopes, and fears, mixed with promise and excitement.

My exam room also serves as my office in the hospital clinic. At the far end, just past the examining table, is a large window with a fifth-floor view of the neighborhood and the two multi-family triple-deckers whose owners seem determined to hold on despite the encroachment of hospital buildings and parking lots. This window gives the room an unusual brightness every season, particularly on spring mornings. My new patient had chosen the metal chair whose bent rods and plain plastic seat and back offered, really, just the ideogram of a chair. This uncomfortable seat does not give the exam room a sense of well-being. I'd recently thought of bringing in a chair from home, my mother's old chair, which my wife had reupholstered in maroon velvet for my birthday. But I hadn't gotten around to it. On the wall behind the patient's chair is a large photograph of vines that my brother-in-law, an artist, had computer-manipulated into the shape of a man kneeling. There are books on the shelves above my desk—textbooks about renal and heart disease, dermatology primers with pictures of common eruptions, guidebooks for how to examine the knee and the shoulder—but I have no pictures of my children under glass, no diplomas in thin black frames on the walls; I've never liked that. Along the opposite wall, there is a small chrome sink next to which I keep square packages of bandages, paper-doll white, and cellophaned rolls of gauze in perfect soft cylinders along the back of the counter. The cabinet above is a cave of supplies, sticks, scalpels, and screw-lid cups hiding in the dark in undisturbed neatness, nothing loose, shaggy, or irregular.

By 11:00 A.M. on that Wednesday, I had already seen three patients, listened to their uncertain stories, examined them, come up with plausible explanations for their symptoms, tried to bestow comfort, and made plans to see them again. I am an internist, a doctor for adults with heart disease, high blood pressure, headaches, hepatitis, and other ailments and illnesses. I take histories and perform physicals. Taking a medical history has a discipline to it, but it's also like listening to gossip where the only topic is the patient who tells stories about herself. On the other hand, the physical, examining a vulnerable and tender body, trying to know its secret past of wounds and scars is exhausting. Physicals confirm histories, but also provide information that patients can't, or won't, communicate. Of course, what doctors don't know about patients, after an hour, even after a year of providing care, is endless. Too often, we are wholly unprepared for what we learn along the way.

What patients don't know about me might be vaster but matters not at all. They *expect* to know little; few ever ask if I have children (I do) or where I went on vacation (I rarely leave home for more than four days), or even where I'd trained, my history of successes and failures. In my twenty years of practice, it has been the rare patient who mentions that they know I am a writer, even though several of my books are for sale in the hospital gift shop.

When I look at patients, I immediately wonder, where, physically, the damage is. Although she was dressed like a teenager, Ms. Lucy Fields had turned twenty-nine recently—her date of birth was stamped on the upper-right corner of her purple chart, which lay open on my desk. She looked healthy—there were no physical signs of illness. Her mouth had a determined shape.

"Can you tell me a little about yourself?" I asked.

Sitting sideways, studying the back of my dark-stained office door and giving me only her profile, she shifted on the metal chair, keeping her feet tucked. She had put her tiny black purse, a white paper coffee cup, and a blue plastic bag with a drawstring on the floor beside her chair. Pretty with her long, black hair that she parted in the middle and pale blue eyes, she was not pretty enough to create envy among the nursing assistants who were known to judge each of my patients. She looked like a girl I went to high school with who always covered herself densely in layers. There is often something in a patient's character or looks or choice of words that binds me to them from the start. Without this connection, I am just a man in a white costume, and they are merely strangers asking me to guarantee they'll live forever.

"I'm tired, I use a lot of Vicodin, and somewhere, deep in the back of my mind, for some reason I still believe that I could have a meaningful life, maybe do something valuable."

This was a bold and risky statement. She couldn't find it in herself to look at me, but I could tell she was ready to talk at length if I made myself available. I could see that there were huge forces at play for her. She was holding herself back from saying too much too quickly despite her opening statement; she didn't want to make a mistake; she wanted a place in my "program." She was wearing two silver and two blue bracelets on her left wrist that made the sound of wind chimes when she reached down and lifted the cup of coffee to her lips.

In 2008, Vicodin was the most prescribed medication in the United States—far surpassing penicillin, Lipitor, and Prozac—a pill chemically related to the opiates (also called narcotics) morphine and heroin. It is offered by internists for back strain and by dentists for toothache, by surgeons postoperatively for incisional throbbing and by emergency room doctors for kidney stones and fractures. Plenty of people use Vicodin legitimately for pain. Occasionally, people who are prescribed Vicodin (or one of its medical opiate relatives, Percocet, codeine, or OxyContin) find that the narcotic not only takes away acute pain, but after only a dose or two helps in unexpected ways. Vicodin gives some users energy while it makes other users feel calm. I had recently seen an exhausted new mother who was given the drug after a hemorrhoidectomy; she was bathing the baby three times a day. These unanticipated gratifications sometimes lead to problems, dependency, and then addiction.

Eleven million Americans take opiates for nonmedical, recreational purposes. Some start with a doctor's prescription, others first try an opiate as a party drug—nothing any more scandalous than marijuana. Most partyers use it once or twice and decide it isn't for them. Others get high and enjoy the euphoric escape. They look for Vicodin the following Saturday night as a reward for working hard, a treat to end the week. There is a spectrum of use (as there is with drinking alcohol), but the ones who make it to my program have been through a definable process: enjoying the Vicodin, having a little fun with it; using it more often, spacing their doses evenly across a weekend day, then evenly across an entire week; then doing anything to get it, having some physical need for it and finding themselves in search of an ever-increasing pile of pills, or moving on to heroin for a bigger, faster feeling. Then gradually they enjoy it less, realizing they can't function without it, but are unable to stop, living with only memories of good times; then with problems mounting, wanting to stop more than anything on earth, disbelieving they ever liked using.

I wondered how Lucy had started, and when, and who else knew she had come to my office.

The "program" she was asking about involves a medication, buprenorphine, which blocks the effects of Vicodin by attaching itself to the same opiate brain receptor. Buprenorphine shares a basic atomic structure with opiates, but does not get the user high because its chemical properties are different. It allows the daily user to escape the urgent, constant, and often destructive calling of his or her habit. It quells the craving. Before buprenorphine, an internist had little to offer an opiate addict. The "program," as far as Lucy knew, was simply my name and office location, which were listed on an Internet site about substance abuse treatment. The site was sponsored by the federal government agency that had granted me permission to prescribe buprenorphine. In early 2005, I was not a "program"—which in its jargon-y sound suggested a twelve-step group—I was simply one of the few physicians in my region specially licensed and trained to treat opiate-dependent patients with buprenorphine. If anything, I was a *de*-programmer, helping a few patients escape the physical and psychic lockdown of addiction. I was also a physician who was skeptical of easy answers, working alone without slogans or a dogma.

Lucy had asked if I had an "opening" because she'd done her research; according to federal law, a buprenorphine provider is allowed to treat only a limited number of opiate-dependent patients at one time. Congress had determined that having a medical practice filled with hundreds of Vicodin, OxyContin, or heroin users was a recipe for diversion—for shoddy prescribing and unavoidable pill sharing among patients—the fastest way to establish a black market of buprenorphine among addicts, and a sure way to promote seepage of this powerful medication into the population at large where nonaddicts might unadvisedly use it for pain and other troubles that might best be evaluated by doctors.

Diverse theories exist about how people become addicts and what should be done to help them. There is far from universal agreement about what constitutes the proper treatment of opiate addicts, how to define treatment success, and how to identify treatment failure—questions that continue to polarize the community of treaters but does little to help the individual doctor in his or her room working with a patient who has found a way to get high.

"What's making you so tired today?" I asked Lucy. What I really wondered was: Why now, why do you want to quit Vicodin now? And what was "tired" code for? But I didn't ask that because addicts hear every judging comment as a reason to walk away. When an addict decides to see a doctor, it is far from decisive. One wrong move on my part and off Lucy Fields would go. She heard my question, then hesitated. I wondered if she thought I was being too personal or too pushy. Perhaps she wasn't used to being observed so closely. My friends say my face is hard to read, that I have an elaborate range of looks, all of which might signal disapproval. I didn't want Lucy to feel defensive. I was not expecting a full account. I didn't know what "a lot of Vicodin" meant yet, but I leaned back in my chair and relaxed.

"What if I tell you that I don't remember what normal feels like? That what *you* feel every day, *I* feel only when I take my pills," she said. She was bowed a little, curled into herself, as if she was expecting something to be thrown at her. It was a posture of no confidence, of unease. "I've done this for so many years I get tired just thinking about it. What if I tell you I'm so tired that I can't get out of bed in the morning, and when I don't get going until the afternoon, I'm sick, and I'm tired of being drug sick. I'm tired of making myself feel better by using."

Her delivery had an almost dreamy quality, as if she was trying not to hear what she was telling me. I've always found that the more emphatically an addict says he or she is ready to quit, the more exuberant the addict is about what he or she might achieve with my help, the less convinced I am that the person will be successful. And the more confident addicts are, the more I worry I'm being manipulated, and that they aren't ready for the hard days ahead.

"I'm just tired," she said.

She looked up for just a moment, regarded me candidly, with a faint smile. Her eyes were alive and intelligent, but she had little sensual presence; she had turned off that part of herself.

I felt a protectiveness toward her.

I looked again for any physical damage as she played with the sleeves of her sweater. Her arms were thin, her skin was not as pale as mine—she obviously tanned easily.

She hadn't yet explained why she had come in *that* morning, that April Wednesday; she had probably been tired for months. My impulse was to make her be more exact, which would oblige her to tell some greater truth about herself. She looked up again quickly.

"I want to go to South Carolina in a few weeks to see my parents. They moved down there a while ago. They used to live here. Now they live in Hilton Head. I haven't seen them in almost two years. It's hard to get away. It's hard to take enough pills on the plane. And it's not worth getting caught."

When patients in pain are prescribed Vicodin, they are expected to take four or six or at most eight pills a day to control their discomfort. By the time most Vicodin addicts come into my program, they are typically using twenty or forty pills a day (needing higher doses to achieve the same effect over time), often spending a few hundred dollars daily on their drug use. In the beginning, a pill or two got them high (or relaxed or energized them, or took away their pain); later, when their bodies adjusted, they needed more for the same effect.

"Do they know you're using?" I asked.

"My mother would say she doesn't. Her powers of denial are really incredibly impressive. If my parents knew about my life right now, my mother would drop dead on the spot."

"But they know you've used in the past."

"They know. But they hate my boyfriend because he's an addict. *He's* the one with the drug problem, they believe. Someone else has the problem, not me. Maybe I used some drugs when I was sixteen, or I had a little trouble when I was twenty-four, they might tell you." She smiled and shook her head in frustration, as if she couldn't believe how blind they were to the facts of her life. She didn't expect me to be sympathetic; she was talking mostly to herself.

All patients invite me to be complicit in their stories, to agree, and to question only as a friend would, without agitation. I am careful not to overstep, waiting to build their trust.

"How could they not know about me, you must be wondering," she asked, as if *I* already knew about her. "I know it sounds improbable. But I let them think it's my boyfriend's fault that I never visit them. You know, I don't know what they believe or how much they just keep quiet to keep the peace. A lawyer and a teacher with a Ph.D., you'd think they'd figure it out."

She had a strange tic. Staring at the back of my door, her eyes would dart at me and she would catch herself, blink and jerk her chin like a hiccup, then look away again, the entire ritual ending with a wince-smile. She never held my gaze.

I wondered what her parents actually knew about her. What had she told them and what had she lied to them about? I also wondered what she would lie to me about. Had she ever had a frank exchange with a doctor since her addiction began? My job is to be sympathetic *and* skeptical. A doctor's mind by nature leaps back and forth between intuition and experience.

Why does addiction intrigue me? To be an addict requires a mental agility and a survivor's creativity that I admire. But there is more to it. I am interested in the opposite side of myself; I fear the appetite that would control me. This young woman, with her good home and professional parents, should have been a model citizen. What happened?

With every drug user I meet, I find myself considering two basic questions: How much do I understand about addiction, and how should I address it? With the next asthma patient, I will have a clear and relatively fixed view of what my care should be and how I explain the disease; the same with my next hypertensive or heart failure patient. Although the medications I use for these conditions might change from year to year, based on updates in understanding of physiology and pathogenesis, I never wonder what asthma and arthritis mean to me. But each addict has a story, and the story is the illness, and what writer can resist that? When a Lucy Fields enters my room, I rethink what it is I am trying to achieve, what I care about and value. I ask myself for the hundredth time: Is addiction a medical illness, a loss of will, an obsessive-compulsive symptom, a character disorder, a spiritual condition, or all of these? Or is it something altogether different?

We are a species that tries to assign blame and admires control. Is addiction a matter of circumstance or weakness? Bad judgment or bad luck? Masochism or machismo? Is the addict someone to be saved or incarcerated? Is she driven by sickness or sin? During my years as a clinician, new drug laws have been passed (three strikes), and new substances manufactured (methamphetamine), and each engendered debate, but altered almost nothing in how I consider these questions. I watch the never-ending array of movies about drug users (*Trainspotting, Down to the Bone, SherryBaby*) and read the newspaper thinking, simultaneously, that what addicts do has nothing to do with me and my wife and kids, but also that addiction has something important to say to and about us.

"For some reason I still believe that I could have a meaningful life." This was the first thing Lucy Fields said and it was probably enough to make me attend to her with an unusual concern and melancholy tenderness. I had certain ideas about addiction and patients' attempts to recover through my "program." I was concerned that medical research, my own research, was perhaps too limited in what it told us about caring for drug-dependent persons. But I also knew how difficult it was to move between ideals and practical ways of assisting the one patient in front of me, how fluid my understanding remained as to how best to help.

Two days each week, I work alongside ten other internists in this clinic. We supply each other with articles to read, and with comfort and courage as we press forward through each day's schedule. We depend on each other for advice and funny stories. We compare and confess our misfortunes. We serve on the same hospital committees, share a weekly seminar, celebrate one another's birthdays and successes. We reveal our particular clinical phobias to one another. My colleague Paul becomes upset whenever he sees above-the-knee amputations, even those that are well healed; he says they remind him of his grandfather. I can barely tolerate the sound of retching. And when we bump into each other among all the commotion and small emergencies of everyday practice, we invite each other into our patient dramas. Then we return to our own rooms, cautiously, like men and women in hiding. At least once a week, I am grateful for a colleague's instruction on something I've forgotten since my training twenty years ago, the proper examination of an ankle, the exact sensory distribution of a lumbar nerve. We share the craving for the company of illness because it offers us the opportunity to feel useful. We get along well, I like to think.

During the remainder of my week, I work in another office in another building, conducting research on addiction. It is clinical research, and therefore does not involve experiments with DNA or cells or mice. Instead, I work with people, many of whom live in the neighborhoods around the hospital, who use chemically active substances. Over the years chemists have determined that there are families of addictive drugs: alcohol, nicotine, stimulants, hallucinogens, marijuana, and, finally, opiates such as Vicodin, my main interest. These drugs are characterized as addictive when lab animals self-administer them to the brink of unconsciousness in a remarkably specific and reproducible way.

The human brain, with its billions of neurons, doesn't have particular cell clusters that constitute an alcohol center, a nicotine center, or an opiate center, but it does have a reward pathway, a particular set of neuronal connections that can be turned on by multiple substances and behaviors that provoke good feelings. Each drug family has its own special dangers when consumed (headaches, heart attacks, delirium), but users rarely take these into account because their main goal is to administer pleasure.

A lot of my time is spent writing proposals to the federal government to study particular clinical aspects of addiction, and to receive grant funding from the National Institutes of Health if my scientific peers believe my ideas are worthy enough to help addicts. My salary is primarily derived from these grants, plus a certain amount from seeing patients in my clinic office; the majority of them do not use drugs illicitly and remind me how addiction is different from other medical conditions. I recruit drug users through newspaper advertisements, posters, in emergency rooms, and through word of mouth—and have, over the past two decades, interviewed thousands about the quantity and frequency of their drug use, their sleep and moods, their criminal pasts and physical disabilities, their families and sex lives. I usually pay study participants for their time—and addicts have plenty of ways to spend their money—so I have no trouble finding study participants. I attempt to understand why some became infected with HIV or other viruses, and I want to learn how and why some addicts change their self-injurious behaviors. I try to assist them in finding a more merciful existence. I publish articles in scientific journals—reasonable, sensible articles about risk and risk-taking. When I take on a patient like Lucy Fields, who was not enrolled in one of my studies, I think about what I've learned and researched and read, and I make an effort to apply it in the clinical setting.

I live in the city where I work, and outside the hospital I see things that might be addiction related—young men punching each other in the face, a woman talking to herself in a doorway, a man on the sidewalk in front of the convenience store with blood streaming from the scabs on his legs. The bleeding man perturbs me; the psychotic woman in the shadows saddens me. I make lists of what could be wrong with them, but I do so to prevent the feelings from taking me over, because outside the hospital, I am not fearless nor particularly altruistic. I do not go out into the destitute corners of my hometown to rescue the drug users in collapsed buildings and abandoned churches. I sleep on a soft bed; I rest after dark. I eat chicken sausage and white beans rather than going out into the night to find lost and starving souls whom I could bring in and help. I hope that my clinic exam room is a refuge for some addicts who find their way to me, but off-duty, I am essentially selfish. My mission, my purpose, is not a life of self-sacrifice—I see patients, I perform my scientific studies, I write books, I am a father and husband. Outside of my office, at home, I work to simplify my life, or create a simple way of seeing the world. But in my examination room on the fifth floor of the Ambulatory Care Center, everything is complicated, or at least I tell myself that.

As Lucy's internist, I wanted to manage her overall health, and I knew that at some point, if she didn't flee, this would involve helping her identify, manage, and master the tyranny of her dangerous, destabilizing needs.

"Do you have a ticket to South Carolina yet?" I asked her.

I thought again about what she'd said about her parents' knowledge of her drug use: *"You'd think they'd figure it out."* I was sure that during her years of Vicodin use, she'd never gotten to many sensitive subjects in her conversations with them, subjects that universally went along with heavy narcotic use: sex, morality, crime, dubious ethics. I thought of how secretive my own teenaged sons had become, out at night, in cars, with their own dark reasons for doing things. What did I know about them? No matter how adept I was at hearing their sighs, reading into their monosyllables, interpreting their moods, gestures, and sounds and nonsounds—did I really know when they felt defeated or hopeless?

"Not yet, but I have to get out of here. Even though it won't exactly be a holiday in South Carolina, I like the heat, and I can probably sit by the pool all day. But I know it won't be easy to spend four days with them. My mother will ask where I'm working and I'll tell her I just quit my job, and she'll say, 'Why don't you call your college alumni association and let them help you find a new one. Maybe you'll meet a nice lawyer.'" She laughed and took another sip of coffee. "That's a joke. Maybe he could represent me."

"You need a lawyer?"

"Not yet."

"Did you just quit your job?"

"A while ago."

"What were you doing?"

"Working in a Laundromat. The perfect job for the graduate of an elite college, don't you think?"

Her rhetorical question let me know that she had judged herself and that she didn't need to hear from me. Delivering herself into my care was difficult, but she would try to be a reliable narrator, and she wasn't going to deny who she was. She had the sensibility and style to pull it off. She was letting me know that she was taking a long and winding path toward something honest, even if, at times, she was likely to trivialize and deflect.

"What do you know about buprenorphine?" I asked.

Developed in the 1970s, buprenorphine had only been approved as a medication in 2003. Part of my research work has been to study buprenorphine, keeping data on every patient I've seen since 2003. What I know is that only 60 percent of my patients who take buprenorphine are still on it six months after starting; the rest have dropped out of care, nearly always returning to the drug that brought them to me. Is 60 percent retention a good outcome or a poor one? How do I compare with other doctors who treat opiate dependence? There is no way to compare because most clinicians, working alone in their offices, do not systematically collect and monitor data about how their patients do. It is shocking how few drug treatment programs can even offer complete and reliable statistics to the inquisitive consumer. There is no incentive, no requirement, for any program to keep figures—let alone release them to the public—and without the facts there is no reason to admit to anything but success.

"I know that I bought one bupe pill on the street a few weeks ago and it gave me a day off from chasing down Vicodin," Ms. Fields said. "Not that I have a lot of trouble maintaining my supply."

Instead of getting up and walking around, she used the metal-armed chair as a gymnast would use parallel bars, bracing her thin arms to lift her light body into the air and adjust it, never facing me but keeping turned sideways toward the door.

"Once we decide to start you on this medication, we'll be seeing each other quite a bit. You'll need to come in to see me two or three times a week for the first few weeks, then less and less often if all goes well. I'll want to see how you're doing, and in the beginning, I'll make sure we have the right dose so that you're comfortable. We'll talk."

"I like to talk. I'm talkative." She looked very sweet, and slightly dispirited.

I smiled. I liked that she liked to talk (because it isn't true of me), that she was not overly earnest, that she was funny and self-mocking. I could be her straight man. I prefer to do the questioning. I am most comfortable in this conventional medical role with its restricted emotional tone, and I appreciate patients who run through their charged lists of complaints and are not unhappy when I ask a few questions, give short answers, and mostly listen. Is this part of what attracted me to medicine, or did it only grow out of my years in this room, where my feelings are so often half-hidden or contained when I deliver good and bad news every day?

If I am addicted to something, it is my need to ask questions.

I have an unquenchable urge to delve, to draw things out of patients, to hear secrets, to hear everything. I like knowing secrets; not to know them is to miss a patient's life. I have difficulty with patients who are restrained or nearly silent. Plenty of the people who come in are surly and are in no mood to do more than list their symptoms. Others are unable to describe how they feel in more than a few words. Some patients are just naturally private.

Medical offices are demoralizing. Disheartened air is still left in the room by the last patient. Often addicts arrive and don't really want their lives changed—they hold on to the belief that maybe their lives are okay the way they are. I have to capture them quickly. They have to be convinced by my conviction and full attention, even when they aren't ready to change. Some addicts just want the next prescription and nothing more. They are eager to go. Some expect me to ask them questions—they have been to plenty of counselors, psychologists, and social workers over the years and are used to giving a little conversation in exchange for their medication.

But some addicts simply want a medical visit that allows them a chance to explain themselves free of authoritative comments and judgments. If I didn't listen, it would be a violation of responsibility and trust. I ask questions because it's my job—the new medical culture encourages internists (not only psychiatrists) to enter the worlds of patients, to absorb their contradictory, resonant stories of illness, to learn their ordeals, strengths, and psychological responses. But I also listen because I have a need I don't understand.

"At each visit—and I'll tell you the schedule in a few minutes after I get through some more screening questions—I'll ask if you're still using Vicodin, and I hope you'll tell me the truth. But I'll also be collecting urine and sending it to the lab to check what you have in your system and confirm what you say."

Before Lucy arrived, I had already seen three patients, each with very different problems than hers—and had enjoyed the morning's successes. My first patient was ninety-five years old and was feeling so well she had decided to move out of her daughter's house and into a place of her own. The second, a tiny man in his fifties, arrived, as always, with his wife and talked about his heartburn and his sweaty palms and how little he ate (his fingers moved in circles to demonstrate the portion sizes) in order to lower his blood pressure, which I'd told him was elevated. These small victories, holding off the inevitable decline of old age and chronic disease, are the satisfactions of an internist's work life. The third patient was a man of sixty with a burning along his lower posterior ribs that I diagnosed as shingles, herpes zoster, a recurrence of the chicken pox he'd had as a five-year-old. Offering a simple and usually effective treatment—antibiotics—for his obvious discomfort put me in a good mood.

My nine daily office hours are like a baseball game—they are innings, segmented, discrete. One after the next, they allow pauses and changes of thinking, arguments and counterarguments, different pitches. To a great degree, I have come to depend on the one-on-one orderliness of medicine in a room surrounded by property and possessions that are mine but not mine. I move through my small world efficiently. I appreciate surprises, although I don't like all of them. In my forty-fifth year when I met with Lucy, I was still surprised that both my parents were dead, and that my older son would be leaving for college in five months. But years with patients have convinced me that everything is possible. Decades past residency training, I believe it is even possible to strike the right note and help most patients who see me as I am, with a scar above my eyebrow and my hair buzz-cut. Still, I wonder if they remember what I look like when they leave my office? Do they think about something I said? Anything I said? Is it easy to keep me distinct from anyone else who provides them service once or twice a year?

I needed to know certain things about Lucy that would influence whether I would give her buprenorphine. This would help me determine if it was the right medication for her—and how we would proceed. I needed to know, for example, if she used any other addictive drugs.

"The medication buprenorphine blocks the effects of Vicodin and any other narcotic you might be taking, as you know, but it doesn't block cocaine. Do you use cocaine?"

Buprenorphine is not a substitute for cocaine—there is no comparable medication treatment for cocaine and doctors are pretty much incapable of affecting how patients use cocaine, so patients who used Vicodin *and* cocaine rarely stick around my office for treatment. If Lucy was a regular cocaine user, I would probably not treat her with buprenorphine.

"I used it a few times about ten years ago."

"But not recently."

"Not at all."

Did I believe her? I've found that even patients who invent their histories eventually disclose the truth if they stick around.

"Do you drink alcohol?"

"Not anymore. I used to, quite a bit." These preliminaries seemed new to her, as if she hadn't visited a doctor in a while.

"When was your last drink?"

"Over a year ago."

"Do you smoke?"

"Cigarettes?"

"Cigarettes. You can also tell me about marijuana."

"A pack will last me three days."

Every survey ever done, including my own research, says that 95 percent of opiate users smoke cigarettes. Part of the reason for this may be that nicotine is a sweet reminiscence for adult opiate users because nicotine was usually the first psychoactive drug many of them used as kids; or possibly nicotine primes the brain for opiates, activating similar cell signals or networks; or maybe cigarettes, begun early, are particularly difficult for opiate users to quit—for both biochemical and social reasons—harder even than opiates themselves. Many opiate-dependent patients hold on to cigarettes as the last, most acceptable vice, even in a world of smoke-free bars, restaurants, and offices.

"No marijuana, though," she added.

"Do you see any other doctors, or take any other medicines?"

"No."

"Is it possible that you're pregnant?"

"Not a chance. My relationship with Brian is about drugs, not sex. We haven't had sex in five months."

"Brian is your boyfriend?"

"The guy I'm with."

Whatever the problems with Brian, whether she was in love with him or not, I could tell the relationship still had a hold on her life. I knew I would learn more about Brian when I heard more about her day-to-day situation.

"Do you have any children?"

"God, I hope not. No, I don't."

A medical license is a license to ask questions. Ordinary conversation disappears quickly in my office. Business has to be taken care of. There is a need to keep up a medical patter so that silent moments do not become unbearably awkward. But unlike in my clinical research studies, which depend on structured lists of questions, asked identically from one participant to the next ("When you shoot heroin, and when the needle is in your vein, do you pull back on the plunger to mix some of your blood into the solution before re-injecting?"), my work in this exam room is less exact. I do not read questions from a page; I trust that I will eventually learn what I need to know. With patients, I get to ask questions like I did as a kid, a near constant battery of whats and whys and hows. I never know what the answers might be until another patient confides his or her story: the widow with the hairy upper lip and sweet powdery smell who had escaped the Armenian genocide; the middle-aged man with cerebral palsy who lived with his mother and visited prostitutes. Each story is like being handed a rescue note: smuggle this out, it's all that's left of me.

"When did you start using?" I asked her.

"Vicodin, or anything?"

"Whichever you want to tell me about first."

"My mother still says, 'You were a happy child.'" Her mouth twisted in contempt, as if this were the most ridiculous thing she had ever heard. "I wasn't a happy child. I was a *miserable* child. I tried alcohol first, like most kids do. When I was thirteen, my father got this bottle of gin as a gift. I found it, emptied the gin into my own bottle, and replaced his with water. He never drank, so he didn't notice. I took the bottle to a friend's house and we drank the whole thing in one night. I threw up eight times on the walk home. But I loved the feeling enough that soon I was drinking every weekend. Then we started drinking Robitussin for the dextromethorphan. That was a good buzz. It was so good, I figured everyone did it. At fourteen, I got weed, which I'd heard you didn't get high from the first few times, and I was so determined to get high I just sat in my room night after night, smoking, until I did. That year, the police came to our house to interview me and my parents. Someone had told the police that I was a drug dealer—they'd searched my locker. I wasn't a dealer; I never have been a dealer. This boy told them I had sold him marijuana—he actually stated a dollar amount. He was making the whole thing up. I'd *given* him some pot, not sold it to him. But I denied it. I remember the sergeant tricked me, though. He said, 'So you're not a dealer, but have you ever done drugs? I won't tell your parents, this is confidential. I can't arrest you for using.' I felt I had to give him something. I said I had used acid twice in the past, and I made up some dates that he wrote on his pad. The next day he called my mother and read her what I'd said to him. My parents immediately grounded me for a month. But of course the next day my mother said, 'Get the hell out of the house, I'm sick of you moping around.' I was a teenager, after all, and nobody can stand teenagers, especially when they're just sitting around."

Lucy laughed, and I could see she liked to laugh.

"I think my mother knew there was a problem on the day I took the SATs. When I was at the test, she cleaned my room and found my gin bottle and the Robitussin and all my smoking equipment. She had lined them up on the dining room table when I walked in. My grades had suffered a little, but not much; I was still in honors classes, and I ended up doing well on the SATs. She sent me for counseling to this weird woman who canceled half her appointments with me, and who eventually told my mother that I didn't have a problem. She was completely incompetent. She was probably an addict herself."

Lucy giggled and pulled her legs tighter underneath her. Doctors, trained in the science of cause and effect and explicable physiology, like to apply a simple directionality to addiction, a single moment, an event, a coherent reason to explain what happened to Lucy. Doctors like single explanations because they promise the possibility of a straightforward remedy.

"My friends started drinking cough syrup the same day I did, but they weren't in trouble with the cops six months later, and they aren't taking Vicodin fifteen years later. That fact at least suggests that there's something in my brain that's not in everyone's. My parents still talk like half my life didn't happen. They know the facts, but they like to pretend that I've had a minor, fifteen-year blip, a Vicodin here or there on this smooth ride to twenty-nine. Who can answer that? The day my mother dropped me off at college, I brought ten quarts of liquor, acid, and weed. I couldn't wait for her to leave, so I could start using again. There's never been a drug I didn't like."

She was no longer giggling. When she finished talking, I realized I knew something about her early drug history, even though she hadn't yet told me how she started with Vicodin.

Any doctor working in an American city at this time is going to face the issue of addiction. We live in the age of addiction. Addiction to chocolate and exercise and shoes and love. Addiction to soap operas, to danger and anger, to golf and the stock market, gambling and cheating. Addiction is the disease of wanting more. More is always better; more becomes necessary. The "more" disease is about impending deprivation. It combines a fear of being without with the sense of never having enough.

Almost anything can be the object of addiction, and most people are a little addicted to something. "Everyone's looking for a fix" was the first line of a nutrition column in a women's magazine I'd once seen lying open on my nursing aide's desk. *Fix* is a drug word that also means "solution." *Everyone*, the new belief. The language of addiction has permeated into the diet columns.

Lucy was college educated, seemingly good-natured, girlish with a broad smile; the daughter of upper-middle-class professionals, she had thick hair and wrists that were pale and thin. Her addiction involved Vicodin, which in the strangely hierarchical thinking of opiate addicts is considered less serious than Oxy-Contin or heroin. "There are worse drugs out there," reported one of my opiate-dependent patients. But maybe not for Lucy. Her intent, starting at age fourteen, was to be a drug *user*, not an addict. Like any addict, she probably still believed she could use Vicodin for just one more day and then could stop.

Fifty years ago, she would have entered a psychiatric hospital for six months to quit her opiate use. Now she could see an internist and receive a prescription for buprenorphine, and no one would even know.

I like the word *addict*. The medical literature of the past decade mostly stayed clear of it, because some medical journal editors believed "addict" was derogatory and could be read as code for underclass, someone who is disobedient and insubordinate. *Addict* is not an empowering word; it is censorious. Addicts are cultural exiles, violators of deeply held social norms. Strangely, the noun "addict" is pejorative, while the adjective "addicted" is not. "Addicted" is more widely used because it connotes one's physical dependence on a substance. The medical literature, focusing on the physiological, prefers the term drug "dependent" to drug "addicted" to characterize patients who use opiates daily, but in a prescribed, regularized manner for diagnosable, painful conditions. My patient Mary, with colon cancer in her liver, used high doses of morphine every day; she was dependent on opiates, and if I didn't refill her prescription she would go into opiate withdrawal. I use the word *dependent* to distinguish patients like Mary from patients like Lucy, who used opiates compulsively, with a narrowness of interest in anything but Vicodin, which occupied and preoccupied her consciousness until she was unable to see the increasing risk and damage.

The word *addict* is an unscrubbed description, unsentimental; nonideological, it captures a feeling of societal disregard. I find myself using it because it is simple, down-to-earth, outwardly accepting, but privately judging and portentous. It captures the antisocial aspects of addiction, the voluntary, indulgent craving, the disinterest in antidotes. When a patient calls herself an addict, she is honoring her reality—hands and neck wet with craving, wanting to get high so badly and believing she'll die if she doesn't—and establishing the difficulty of abolishing it. One Vicodin user can call another *addict*, but for a doctor to introduce the term is to go beyond the bounds of civil conversation. In the office, *addict* is like a curse word, impersonal, but also cruelly personal.

To at least one of my colleagues, addict was shorthand for angry and disengaged. He found himself using it automatically around me when he assigned a patient he didn't particularly like over to my care for the weekend. My colleague said nothing more than "This one's a thirty-five-year-old cocaine addict in the hospital with chest pain," permitting my subconscious to do the work. He was telling me he'd handed off a patient who was ragged, dangerous, and hopeless—someone who stole from his parents and abandoned his kids. My colleague figured that it would be difficult, once I heard the word *addict*, to turn it off, and that I should feel free to treat this patient callously, if necessary.

A patient once told me how he could spot another addict on the street. He said it's all in the eyes. Not only are the pupils tiny, the eyes follow every passing car. They watch carefully, hungrily. Each car that slows down holds a potential customer or a potential vendor.

Movies have taught us to recognize addicts. We notice their

faces: scratched, acned, pocked. We look at their eyes and recognize them at first sight no matter how they try to cover it up. In movies, the addict's face has a meanness when he is around drugs; you can't miss it. These scenes are filmed in bathrooms or doorways or alleys, always in darkness. To catch sight of a heroin addict in the act is confusing, mysterious, slightly awe-inspiring. *Everyone's looking for a fix.* As moviegoers, we accept the addict's routine helplessness. We believe we can apprehend how quickly he'd fallen, how desperate she was. Movies have taught us the cold hard dynamics of the junkie's transaction. We gape at the addict's tiny tragedy with unembarrassed fascination. We notice his expression: blurred, frozen jawed, suppressing a moment's rage.

Even after years at my job, it was difficult to use the word *addict* as my colleague used it and not think of someone aimless, indifferent, sullen. Red-eyed and numb-fingered, the addict in the movies lived a makeshift life among spare furnishings: a table for cards, a bed with one cigarette-burned blanket, a refrigerator maddeningly empty. High, riding a bus, he seemed dead, abandoned, but he could come alive at any moment, crazed, disordered, dangerous, cold and acquisitive, unsentimental and nearly indestructible. He nodded off and startled awake in a series of death and resurrection exercises while we watched him out of the corners of our eyes.

We wanted to yell, "Just stop." But of course addicts couldn't just stop, or wouldn't. Nothing could stop them. While we might sympathize, we also despised them. Addicts were the too-easy targets of a too-obvious system of disapproval.

There was another movie version. In this one, the addict is Ray Charles or Charlie Parker, Sid Vicious or Kurt Cobain, Jim Morrison or one of the legions of artists we might admire. The legend of the creative addict is tenacious. The artistic professions, and music in particular, seem to invite narcotics. It is part of the territory, the persona. The creative addict is a seeker who aspires to a higher level of experience and consciousness. Drug use began as a search: for rapture, for the rebirth of feeling. He had had to make a choice between naïveté and madness and he had chosen to access visions that the unaltered brain could not. The artist occupies himself with his private interests as if he is alone in the world. He delights in suffering. When he is sober, he wants to be high; when high, he wants to be sober. He is tortured, attractive, deep. Drug use is a sign of passion, and passion alters personality, making everyone more alive. Passion hypnotizes with the need for release, eyes rolling back in cruel pleasure.

Even when each day became torment and demonic possession, there was meaning to the addict-artist's search. We knew he was surrendering his will to addiction in order to let creativity shine through. Drugs were liberating before they became confining, before he became grim and easy to deplore. Passion's goal is joy, but passion could also become imbued with a sense of desperation. The addict, alert to his darkest secrets, reminds us of our own worst anxieties, the primacy of our desires. But the addict, the wholly passionate one, is eventually incapable of running his own life; addiction compromises autonomy. The artist eventually becomes distracted, anesthetized, submerged, unable to work or function. What seems like a potent rage to live becomes suicidal. This is the movie's arc. When passion becomes simplified to addiction, it is unidimensional. The artist comes to believe that addiction has chosen him. Out of control and compulsive, he loses the normalcy of his life, his concern for kids and parents and friends. He reforms or dies.

If we are romantic, we believe the addict is after transcendence.

If we are realists, we believe they are simply escaping. Addiction, as a patient once told me, is actually a fear of life. To go to a movie about addicts is to engage in catastrophe at a distance.

I've spent hours talking to addicts, but I know little of what really goes on in those alleys, cars, and bathrooms. Using the props I've been given by filmmakers and the words I've heard in my office, I imagine in general terms how my patients survive, but it's really nothing more than pure speculation. The sickest parts, the parts that don't make it into the movies, are the parts addicts can't tell anyone, the parts they aren't ready to tell me until I've known them for a year or more.

Prescribing buprenorphine is a way of seeing addiction close-up. It's also a way of knowing that each patient's personal catastrophe *can't* be easily cured, even as I approach with clemency and nonjudgment in my heart.

Why am I interested in addiction? Why can't I politely agree that drug addicts are basically criminals? The answer is that my heart has always leaped when anyone, in a movie or in my office, escapes—from poverty, from a bad marriage, from bad habits like Vicodin. I am an optimist. I believe in the saying "There is no such thing as bad weather, only the wrong clothes."

From my fifth-floor office window, I can see much of the southern part of the city. The hospital campus fills the foreground, its crowded oil-stained parking lots inside standard, chest-high, diamond-wire fencing; narrow sidewalks leading to wheelchair ramps that enter low brick buildings; slow-moving vehicles, haltingly trying to read signs with arrows in order to locate destinations for pickups and drop-offs; the universe of the ill, each patient in peril every day, wearing velour beach robes and hair rollers and wraparound sunglasses and cowboy boots, struggling with bags, limping and puffing. From this vantage, there are telephone lines everywhere, crowded as needlepoint, nearly obstructing the view, carrying X-ray images and calls to loved ones far away, and digitized blood test results and wirebound viruses. Encircling the hospital property two blocks away, a fallen neighborhood—abandoned gas stations, vacant lots, small businesses, liquor stores, pawnshops, Dominican churches, and brightly neoned fast-food outlets, set among shabby retail establishments (paints, car batteries for sale), with windows so dirty it was difficult to tell if commerce continues there. But just outside my window, a few holdouts, that pair of triple-deckers with small square lawns, with sheets and towels drying on balconies in the chilly air, where grown children live upstairs and disabled parents down.

Eventually all the patients from the neighborhood, addicts included, make it to one or another doctor in this building. Every day twenty needy people bombard me with stories that are meant to lead to a definite, useful, authoritative conclusion. These stories are offered with a clear and practical directive: cure me.

Lucy Fields bent over and picked up the tiny black purse she'd laid beside her chair. She held it up toward me, hidden in her grip. "My mother gave me this purse two years ago, the last time I saw her. Ridiculous little feminine thing. It's cute, but now I have to carry a separate bag so I have room for a notepad and the book I'm reading. My purse won't hold anything more than aspirin and a checkbook. Not that I have a checkbook, or even a savings account at this point."

"Do you read a lot?"

"I'm always reading a novel." When she smiled, the corners of her eyes crinkled.

Maybe this was the true source of my interest in helping her.

Maybe this other habit of hers, books, which very few patients carried into my office.

"What are you reading these days?"

"Dickens. *Hard Times*. I've read every Dickens twice at least."

I remembered *Hard Times*: all the children innocent and pure, every adult redeemable.

"When did you finish college?"

"About eight years ago. I graduated, but I have no idea how. Yes, I do. I was always good at school if I paid attention. Actually, even if I didn't.

"After nearly twenty years of going to school, I don't even know what I like to do, or how I would know what kind of career I want. Career. Listen to me talking about a career. I haven't held a job for more than two months. I *must* be preparing to visit my mother. I actually envy people whose families are without expectations. My family's expectations would be unreasonable in even the best circumstances. And today's visit with you, no offense, does not signify the best circumstances."

"What do they expect?"

"It's pretty specific: social status, education, income. Because of the life they've had, it translates into educational and economic accomplishment. My parents had academic aspirations for me since I showed promise at age six. They still think I should be in school. They're bourgeois, but basically my mother wants to see that I'm not self-destructive. She has a lot of her happiness invested in me. I don't know if I'd want children. How can anyone make that investment?

"My younger sister, I don't know if she'll ever have a problem in life. Actually, she probably feels ignored. Growing up, all the attention was on me. It's still on me. It's been on me since age thirteen for bad reasons."

"She doesn't use drugs?"

"She's a normie. That's what I call her. Her life is normal, like most people's."

I wanted to tell her and each of that day's patients that it had been a difficult year for me, too. My mother died of cancer, slowly. A year before, on Christmas day, a Thursday morning, she called me by pushing the redial button I had circled on her phone. She said she couldn't get out of bed; her back had "locked up." The day before she had been active, again rearranging her paintings among the hooks I had sunk eight years before into the soft walls of her apartment six blocks from my home. At eighty-one years old, my mother had a terrific capacity to absorb pain, so whatever was pinning her to the bed was sure to be bad. I met the ambulance crew at the front door of the assisted-living facility where I had moved her and led them upstairs with their stretcher. Her two rooms had a fecal smell. She was chipper until they tried to lift her. In the emergency room, the first X-ray revealed a collapsed lumbar vertebra. The second, of her chest, showed a large tumor in her right lung. No treatment was recommended for the cancer other than analgesia.

Every day until she died, she was in pain in her single bed, despite the morphine and massages the visiting nurses gave. On the worst days, I thought of asking one of my patients to buy me some heroin to see if it would work any better than the standard stuff, although I knew it wouldn't. Heroin is just an opiate cousin to the morphine she was getting, but it has a magical name and, according to connoisseurs, is considered the best option for unforgiving pain.

Although it had driven me crazy for years, my mother's dementia now proved valuable to her: it defeated any possible memory of yesterday's pain. Each day's suffering was new; each day she wondered why her back hurt. She had no idea how long she had been in pain. She endured illness, she scowled through it, but she wasn't scared of tomorrow. For no good reason, I rooted for her to survive the devastation longer than I should have.

I stayed home from work for only a day after the funeral. I forced myself to remember what I could of my boyhood feelings and of the brave talk she and I had after my father died when I was thirteen. I'd felt cheated over a lifetime without him. There were times when I understood nothing of my own life, but one thing I knew was that I had to get back to work as soon as possible. Medicine in its proper sequence—history, physical, thinking, and only later, feeling—was a relief during those first weeks of grief over her death.

Lucy asked: "I'll take *some* responsibility for things I did when I was thirteen, but I was *thirteen,* so how much responsibility can I take?"

She had no illusions about her youth. It had been broken, bad humored. She had idealized nothing as it receded into the past. The tone of her voice betrayed a sense of anguished desolation.

"I know I can't be held responsible for everything I did. I just can't. But when I think like that, I feel bad for myself. Poor me. I was afflicted and nobody helped me. But the way I used alcohol and drugs, the way they immediately affected me, tells me I had a disease, and no one will ever convince me otherwise."

The most compelling evidence that addiction has physiological roots is the way an addict's body responds differently to its drug of choice than the nonaddict's. It was not a matter of knowing how or when to stop; once an addict starts, stopping doesn't feel like an option.

"How did you start with the Vicodin?"

"I stole it from my mother when she was sick with cancer. Lymphoma. A lump in her neck. She almost died from a reaction to the chemotherapy. I was a junior in college, so I didn't see her that much during the worst of it. I was around for a few weeks after she got out of the hospital. She had bottles of pain pills, and she hated taking pills. So I took them. I took a few out of her bottle at first. I got high, but I remember I felt sick. The next day, I went back to school sick, vomiting."

I imagined that outside my office Lucy was on guard, terrified of being found out, used to hiding. But here, she spoke openly.

"Before I got sick I liked the feeling of being sort of asleep while I was awake. So I took a few more each day."

Users have many ways of explaining the beginnings of their problem. She had gotten sick from alcohol and sick from Vicodin and yet continued both. But somewhere before this initial nauseating bodily reaction, the drug of choice always brings a feeling of warmth and protection. *I liked the feeling of being sort of asleep while I was awake.* Nearly all my patients describe taking drugs as a remedy for some difficulty they didn't realize they had until they felt better.

Before I'd met many addicts, I was skeptical that someone could start abusing narcotics in their thirties or forties even though they'd never had even the hint of a drug or alcohol problem as a teenager. Was it really possible that a thirty-five-year-old woman could be handed a Percocet by a friend to relieve menstrual cramps and a year later be using them not only during her periods, but every day? Could a twenty-eight-year-old lawyer hurt his shoulder building a deck on his house, take one of his buddy's Vicodins, and three years later be swallowing $200 worth of OxyContin daily? I have never had a friend offer me a Percocet for pain. Neither had any of my relatives, or friends, when I asked about their experiences. Are my patients and I really living in such different Americas? Am I in the mainstream, or are they? It is not unusual to learn that an addict's husband has drinking problems, or an older brother "runs with a bad crowd." Often, there is more than a glancing acquaintance with risky behavior. But frequently narcotics are a patient's first and only lifetime vice. Often, I am the first person to know. My patient with menstrual pains hid her addiction from her husband; it was the only thing about her he didn't know.

"I fooled myself into thinking my mother didn't know I'd stolen her pills, but years later she told me she did." Lucy briefly looked up to scan my face to see if I believed her.

"Can we start today?" We were not sitting very far apart. She had a bitter coffee breath. Outside my window, gulls drifting over from the bay jeered. Addicts presume that the day they decide to seek treatment, it will be available.

"Unfortunately, we can't. When you come back from the bathroom, I'll tell you why, but now I need you to give a urine sample so that I have documentation of what drugs you've taken recently and confirm your Vicodin use."

She had the look of a child denied a prize at a party.

When she returned carrying a half-filled plastic specimen cup wrapped in a plastic bag, her expression was bemused, as if she'd learned quite a bit about me in the last half hour and looked forward to what was next. I explained that certain medications have the power to prevent sickness and others can sicken. Buprenorphine has such a powerful affinity for the brain's opiate receptors that when it arrives there, it will displace any Vicodin that is attached. When Vicodin was knocked off Lucy's receptors, her body would go into sudden and severe withdrawal, worse than any drug withdrawal she might ever have experienced. To avoid this, she had to begin the buprenorphine when she was already experiencing the early stages of withdrawal; if she was in mild withdrawal, the effects of the buprenorphine would not be as drastic. Currently, she wasn't in withdrawal—she had taken her last Vicodin a half hour before she arrived—so I couldn't begin her buprenorphine right then. I explained that she needed to plan the timing of her final Vicodin such that she would be uncomfortable, but not quite puking; at that point I would give her the buprenorphine.

Once on it for a few days, she would feel well again. Buprenorphine is a once-a-day pill that releases its synthetic opiate slowly, causing its effect to last for more than a day. It would offer a new equilibrium—not a high, but a release from the physical need to return to the tiring life of Vicodin. I wanted Lucy to start on a Monday, so I could see her several times during her first week on treatment.

"Five days from now?" She was fiercely disappointed. This seemed to confirm some idea she had that I wasn't actually going to help her. She was annoyed. She wanted to start treatment immediately. She was right to think that she could have done what I'd just described at home, on her own. Why was I complicating things?

I tipped my head as if the wait were out of my control. I also wanted her to think about her commitment to joining the "program." Was she willing to see me several times a week for the next month? Once stabilized, was she willing to continue to see me monthly until she'd dealt with the reasons she'd come in, at which time we would talk about stopping the buprenorphine? I wanted her to read everything she could about buprenorphine on the Internet, or in the pamphlets I handed her, which she slid into her blue plastic bag, drawing the string tightly once they were inside.

I wanted her to prepare. The beginning of any medical treatment is the worst. There is confusion and fear. For addicts, the first days are about admitting a history they'd rather ignore. Could Lucy really imagine a life without Vicodin? She would waiver, struggle. The decision to quit never comes easily. She was "tired"; she wanted to "feel normal"; she wanted to visit South Carolina. I did not feel cruel making her wait five more days after she'd been using for five hundred days in a row. She was right to think I was testing to see if she'd come back. Whatever the rituals of her use, they were needful and soothing, and now she would have to figure out how to put them aside.

She didn't protest. She had come in search of salvation, and not all was gloomy. At her next visit, treatment would begin. Once I wrote a prescription for buprenorphine, once my name was on her bottle, we were linked.

"If you'd known it was going to cause all these problems, do you think you'd still like that feeling of being asleep while you're awake?" I asked.

"Yeah, I probably would. I guess that's a sign that I'm in trouble, wouldn't you say?"

For an hour I had been asking myself why she had really come in, and why today—as if there were good reasons and bad reasons for trying to quit Vicodin. Every visit with me going forward would be loaded with misgivings for Lucy, no matter what reason she had come in. Was accurate self-assessment even possible? Didn't addicts bend every truth to appeal to me or to convince themselves? Was there anything more to it than the possibility of a different life?

As she left my office—she walked away quickly, the strap of her tiny purse half an X across her blouse, shoulders hunched, head down, a tall woman in a hurry—I wrote Lucy Fields into my calendar for Monday, April 21, at nine in the morning.

CHAPTER 2

Friday, April 18

Lucy Fields is an exception. Only a small minority of the addicts who come to see me do so with the burden of self-knowledge that they are addicted and want to quit. Perhaps I remember Lucy's first visit so well because my final patient of that week had picked my name from his insurance company's register of internists accepting new patients. He had no idea I was interested in addictions.

When I stepped out of my exam room, he was already waiting for me. He had escaped the grimness that infiltrates all waiting areas. He had not waited for the nurses to summon him; he was making sure he was seen promptly. I had the sense that this patient was competing with the others who had arrived early, demonstrating that he was suffering more than they. He looked to be about my age, and he was clearly eager to be helped. Patients with a fierce need to get better had high expectations of themselves and of me; they worked hard to find and adhere to the recommended treatments. In my practice, assertive self-preservation and perseverance were the best predictors of success. I felt pressured by his stare. Most patients were usually quiet and private until I began the nameless rite of accepting them into the exam room and closing the door. This one had broken rank.

From a distance, the long oval of his face made him appear tall, even though he was under six feet. He had a thin nose, small pouches under his eyes, and his puffy hands bore no rings. His clothes were drab—a striped and hooded sweatshirt, and blue sweatpants that didn't look clean. He had short curly hair and I imagined that when he was a nervous boy, he might have wound each strand around his finger and released its coiled spring. He moved toward my room and toward me. Rather than stopping to greet me, to make eye contact and shake my hand, he disappeared past me. Inside my office, before I'd even introduced myself, he announced, "Doc, I really need something for this pain."

I followed him in and sat at my desk while he leaned against the wall, beginning a detailed account of a car accident six months earlier. He looked around, but not casually, telling me that the emergency room he'd visited said he hadn't broken anything. He believed them but his pain continued, "all over, in my bones, my back mostly." If he'd been sitting, I would have described his behavior as squirming.

He kept talking, barely giving me a chance to interrupt or even slow him down, and he didn't appear to be in terrible pain—no doubling over, no temple rubbing, no grimacing. He was nervous and impatient. He wanted relief, but it wasn't exactly clear what the problem was. He didn't appear emaciated or brittle or weak. I never ask patients to rate their pain, preferring instead to watch and learn what they can and can't do because of it. I was perplexed, unable to judge, at first, the extent of his discomfort. I could think of no immediate link between his relentless and diffuse pain and his accident, and so I began to generate a list of other possibilities: a systemic muscle inflammation, an unusual infection, most likely viral, a rare metastatic cancer.

I am a list maker. Before knowing a diagnosis, I make lists of possible causes along with solutions to a symptom so as to avoid the mindless habit of leaping directly to the diagnosis I see most frequently or have the greatest fear of overlooking. I make lists as a way of preventing the dementia from which my mother suffered during the last five years of her life.

I hadn't answered quickly enough, and with the thin, breaking voice of alarm he said, "Doctor, listen, I really do need something. The sooner, the better."

A reminder, a plea, a command? He had a weak chin. His eyes were dark; they had witnessed an inglorious past.

"Can you tell me your name?" I finally managed.

"Dan," he said, extending his hand and shaking mine roughly. He told me he didn't care what was causing the pain; he just wanted it gone. "I just need something," he repeated several times. His pain had no obvious boundaries, and I guessed that it would not respond promptly to treatment.

"Please, sit down," I offered.

"Not right now," he said. "This pain won't quit."

Listening is what I do for a living, although sometimes I shine a light in a patient's eyes, push a stick into his mouth. A doctor's job is to keep his attention from becoming fractured, confused, weakened. The plotline of illness often involves a maddening

profusion of details, generally offered by the patient with mis-
leading emphases, repetition, and inconsequential turns. Patients
feel there is too much to be said and that it's impossible to say it
all, or clearly.

I could tell from Dan's tone that he expected me to disappoint
or frustrate him, although I hadn't said a word since I'd asked if
he wanted to sit. I was highly aware of his delivery—unusual in
its timing, request, and emphasis—the sidestep of convention by
not waiting for me to begin the questions that would eventually lead to his "need." It was not exactly unsettling to reach the
heart of the visit—pain relief—so quickly, but he was in a hurry
and that was atypical for a patient's first visit. Patients always try
to win my sympathy. To do so, they make every effort to come
across as logical, rational, and measured. But not *this* patient, at
least not at the beginning of this visit; he had other urgent things
on his mind.

He stood over me, no more than two feet away, shuffling, refusing my offer of a chair. Looking up at him was like sitting too close
to the movie screen, a filled-up vision when there was nothing but
film before me. This patient looked well, but he was telling me he
wasn't. The future for a person in pain is always arduous and in-
definite. I wondered if he was standing because being upright was
the most comfortable position. I noticed the way his toes pointed
slightly inward.

For ten minutes, I listened to his description of the rear-ending
accident and the whiplash and the emergency room visit, and the
escalating nature of the pain, and his vision of relief.

Then came three words: "Percocet usually works."

The list of medical possibilities shrank to one.

During a normal day of seeing twenty patients, how many ask
me for a specific medication? There is the occasional insomniac

who has seen a television advertisement for a sleeping pill; there is the person with seasonal allergies, or the astute hypercholesterolemic who has read his *Merck Manual*. My nephews, college kids, are amateur pharmacologists who have grown up not only with direct-to-consumer advertising, but in a magazine world of symptom checklists and a computer culture of online pharmacies. They believe there is a pill for everything; which one to take is a matter of personal choice—a little of this for attention deficits, a little of that for anxiety. But how many patients do I see who actually name the pain pill they prefer?

The central premise of medical training is the paramount importance of diagnosis. It is the centerpiece of faith in the medical process. Diagnosis is illumination; the only hope of cure is knowing what needs to be treated. Diagnosis imposes a right/wrong distinction. The diagnostic "what" is the end result of Sherlockian logic, the central rationalism of the physician's clue following. The doctor in search of a patient's diagnosis must be like Sherlock Holmes, a combination of bloodhound, pointer, and bulldog. When a doctor proves a diagnosis, he or she has provided evidence that reason can triumph over the illogic of illness.

With certain patients, the answer does not matter. Sometimes commitment to diagnosis is too stark, or beside the point. For patients with kidney failure, the original cause of the kidneys' scarring is rarely important (except to warn family members who might have inherited a similar condition); the treatments, dialysis or transplant, are the same regardless of the cause. But when a patient has pain—the most subjective and indisputable of medical complaints—cause matters because it dictates very different treatments.

It seemed unlikely that Dan was using Percocet for legitimate, car-accident-related pain (diagnosis #1), because if he were, wouldn't a doctor already be prescribing it to him? There were other clues. Despite his agitation, he had, after all, named his medication of choice, and he had not asked me to investigate causes or suggest alternative treatments. That left the more likely possibility that Dan was addicted to Percocet (diagnosis #2). His addiction might have begun with a doctor's prescription, perhaps even after an accident, or he might have started Percocet for pleasure. In either case, Dan had become physically dependent on opiates. He would begin to have opiate withdrawal twelve hours after he ran out of his last pill, and I figured from his pointed request that he had come to my office because his supply was low or gone. As soon as pain is announced, the diagnosis becomes subordinate to helping the patient, regardless of the original reason for his or her physical dependence on opiates; this is where the physician's task begins and ends. If Dan's pain did not exist, if this visit was only a means to restock his Percocet collection, then writing him a prescription for Percocet would put me in the role of his accomplice.

I was already thinking of ways I might help him, but I knew it would be difficult to retain his attention. Doctor talk is usually tediously practical, and he wanted something from me.

I considered, for a moment, whether I should simply test my intuition, *"I think you're addicted to Percocet."*

I don't ordinarily ask patients to divulge their secrets right away, even if I sense they aren't telling me the whole story. Would telling him I knew he was dependent on Percocet be an accusation? I wanted to ask: *Are you high or straight?* If I had any hope of helping this man, I didn't want to scare him off. He was used to running, I was sure. Approach slowly, I told myself, hands open and extended, but without revealing the sugar cube he's looking for. I reminded myself: don't ask too much of him too quickly.

Part of me wanted to bully Dan—to provoke a certain kind of response was a familiar urge. When a patient doesn't admit to his problem, a recklessness can grip me. Restraint seems pointless. When the situation is dire, I often feel ready to explode. Each patient's visit has its share of suspense, and not only because I can't anticipate what will come next, but because I need to hold back so many reactions, so many feelings. With Dan, I couldn't wait to react fully, deeply, without restraint. But experience told me that it was too early.

"Please sit. I have a few questions to ask you." He seemed confused by my formality. He had been talking to me as if I was someone he'd known for some time.

I was already planning to refuse his Percocet request. I would claim that I never prescribed narcotics for diffuse body pain, certainly not at a first visit, as if I were just stating the law. *I don't, that's just my policy,* I would claim. I could have saved us both time, and I could have been done with him. But I didn't.

Why? Why did I try to engage Dan of the tapping feet, of the elliptical face and silent curses? I had been told it was impossible to have any meaningful patient-doctor relationship with an addict. But I had come to believe that the only hope was the possibility of establishing one. I pride myself on not being misled by sentimentality, which is to say, I don't believe that with special suffering comes special virtue. Although this may be a morally irresistible connection, it is, as every doctor who works with addicts knows, a misunderstanding, and plays no part in helping any recovery.

Many of the addicts who come to see me claim they began using narcotics to treat the acute pain of a medical condition. One started after sinus surgery, another in the wake of uncontrollable migraines. Hearing these stories made me feel superior, savvier than my doctor colleagues who had naively started these addictions—even in the cases of what sounded like appropriate original prescriptions. Why hadn't they been more careful with what they prescribed? Couldn't they see the risk profile of the particular patient? Of course they couldn't. One percent of American adults have admitted to having tried heroin during their lifetime, but only 9 percent of these individuals used it in the last month, which to me means that though the urge to experiment is not uncommon, lifelong addiction to even this mythically addictive opiate is rare.

My reaction to other doctors' prescribing behaviors is retrospectively skewed. The original treating physician had probably written a perfectly reasonable prescription, strong analgesics for a few days or a week for a believable pain complaint, having no reason to believe this particular suffering patient would have a problem with opiates; the doctor had treated hundreds of other patients in an identical manner and these patients had been fine. Most often the treating doctor never again sees the man or woman who becomes my addicted patient. They have unintentionally tripped a fuse that will explode only months or years later, and they would be appalled if they knew, if they thought they were in any way involved.

Some patients find doctors who unknowingly abet a nascent attraction to narcotics. This or that physician extends a one-month supply of Vicodin, prescribed after the routine repair of a fractured femur, to four or five months, as the young, smooth-talking, well-employed mortgage broker, whose skiing accident caused the broken bone in the first place, comes in for regular follow-ups with persistent pain. Some patients find physicians who ignore what is clearly a pattern of pill-seeking, but this kind of physician—called "croakers" or "script doctors"—are well known to the addicts of any decent-sized city in America.

Over the years, every one of my addicted patients who had received long-term prescriptions from a single provider was reluctant to rat on his or her doctor-suppliers; they wouldn't give names. Did they believe these doctors had been well-wishing and didn't deserve my scorn? Did they believe these doctors had done them a favor and thus deserved loyalty? Did they imagine that someday they might head back to this source and so didn't want to burn that bridge? Even those who blamed these doctors for feeding their problem would not disclose names.

Narcotic addicts who started as teenagers move me in a different way. The average person, the average *doctor,* has little idea how such a life came about. And most young addicts, once grown, willfully refuse to remember the way things were. For those of us who function in the world of straightforward facts, these lives of youthful opiate addiction organized around survival are almost unbelievable.

"So you've decided not to help me," Dan said.

It was a question and a statement rolled into one. His tone was both admonishing and full of derision. He looked me in the eye, challenged me. He feared no one, and apologized to no one. I often think of the exam room as a laboratory—anyone watching would get a strong sense of human behavior under duress. A combination of naked pride and helplessness—announced in a lonely, ordinary, wounded man's voice. That's what it took for Dan to ask for Percocet from me, a stranger in a white coat. I might have defended my interest in him, my decision, in fact, to try to help him, by admitting to an internist's *over*optimism, or else to an addiction specialist's conceit and selfish insistence.

"Look, I've been here for more than fifteen minutes. I need something for my pain. How long am I going to have to wait? And not Tylenol. Something strong."

He said this as if I could pull open a drawer and hand "something" over. When addicted to a narcotic, patients assume that narcotics are everywhere. I could almost hear his cells ticking; he was a Geiger counter detecting imagined opiates. He didn't care if I meant well; he didn't care at that moment what I believed would do him good. Dan wanted the right answer, the right pill, and fast. Like doctors, addicts are really not patient, not even a little. I identified with this wild-eyed man before me: we were both temperamental people who were willing to barge in and demand things from people who would rather not have anything to do with us. I had done it recently with teachers in my son's high school: let's start a school newspaper, would you, my son wants to learn journalism. It will be good for him and good for the school. The difference between Dan and me was that he didn't cloak his demands in self-righteousness.

He put his back firmly against the closed door. Watching him move, I wondered again about the severity of his pain, which I presumed by then was solely due to the early hours of opiate withdrawal. He hadn't cried out or winced. If he had during the first minutes of his visit, I might have been compelled to accept his pain. Screams are incontestable. Screaming is not only a confession that one has lost control, but a way of transferring pain, of giving it to the listener. A scream is an announcement, an acting out, an accusation: you are not doing enough to help me. But Dan had another way of expressing himself that day.

I thought he was simply standing close to my chair, which happened to be near the door, rather than blocking the door. I realized he was in a savage state. To be in pain is to be virtually unconscious, concentrating on the narrowest slice of being. All else is obliterated. Dan was raw, unstable, fragile, exposed. He saw that he was about to lose something (an easy Percocet prescription). He was aware he was living badly, but he didn't care right then. He wanted something from me. He was ferocious and alert; every addict's life comes down to this, and not infrequently.

There is violence inside hospitals, and I am often surprised there isn't more. In my experience it breaks out most often in the emergency room, the airport terminal of the hospital, the site of comings and goings, of transience, the stopover for travelers, the first landing for the already hurt. There is pain and fear, there is the anger and frustration that comes with bad luck's arrival, compounded by the delays—for blood work and X-ray results— where it is clear that the staff is taking care of many people, where you aren't the only one, just the one they are slowest to assist. This feeling of being ignored, the sense that not enough attention is being paid, makes people crazy. There is hugging and laughing in the emergency room, but also pushing and crying. I need to be seen now; I'm the important one. There is anxiety, worsening every minute. Violence soothes panic. Desperation instructs: strike before being struck.

In the hospital—whether it is the emergency department or the clinic—where so many are weak and thin and might never recover, we insist on a kind of normalcy. Doctors, staring at injury and deformity, are models of acceptance. This facade lessens fear. Anyone can get better. The chaos and judgment of the world are not allowed in. Doctors are imperturbable. The hospital is not the same as the world outside. This is why violence is so intrusive.

Mostly, Dan wanted to puncture my pretense of being at ease. Why should I be calm when he was in pain?

Although Dan was nearly my age, I felt like an old man beside him. I felt like a parent. I was an emblem of punitive morality. Although I never thought of abandoning my sons even if they were incapable of following the simplest instruction, even if they tried me with their complicated and distressing problems, and even if they stood over me, misbehaving, I wasn't so absolute about patients.

I was a little frightened by Dan, but mostly I was angry that he was angry, and that we were adversaries, and that he was standing over me—threateningly—at 4:30 in the afternoon. Standing in front of the door was a way to shake me up. He *wanted* to shake me up, take me by the medical shoulders and destroy my elaborate physician's pose. He was making a spectacle, a crisis of the visit. He was the sort of man you wouldn't challenge unless you knew you could get to the door faster than he could. I was sifting and ordering my options, trying to decide what I wanted to do, which is not necessarily the same as doing what should be done. It seemed possible to feel angry and responsible at the same time.

In my mind, I studied the small print of my contract with Dan, looking for a way out of this situation. But there wasn't one. Even if I refused his Percocet request, I was stuck with him for now, unless he bolted, frustrated and miserable, or swung at me. There was a way out for him, but not for me. In this way he had a certain power over me.

The need to deliver him from dishonesty, to have Dan admit that his pain had nothing to do with a car accident six months before, suddenly seemed important.

I made a decision: I would not stand up. I did not need to match him in this way. *I* had all the power. He needed my prescription. Although he may have been holding back an explosion, blocking the door was a device, and a childish one at that. He was trying to speed me along. His foot began to tap again and this tapping told me I was not in danger. I felt badly for him, but I also wanted to make a good showing, to present myself as cool and rational and sympathetic, someone Dan could work with in case the visit turned in another direction, toward honesty.

Outside in the hall, I heard the soft clicking of computer keys. I heard someone calling for a nurse to perform an EKG.

Dan had not yet fled, so I tried to engage him, to draw him out, to learn more about him if he was willing, to treat him humanely, not because I was expected to or should have, not because I agreed to care for every patient who came in with complicated pain issues, but because I wanted to. He was unwell. I did not want to send him off.

"I can't give you any medication until I know a little more about what's going on with you," I said.

I spoke slowly, trying not to patronize him. Condescension when turning down any patient's request is almost inevitable. I heard myself stressing the *can't*. I heard myself trying not to sound urgent, trying to remove the urgency from this visit.

I expected him to explode with disbelief. He couldn't understand what I was there for, what purpose I served, if not to relieve his pain in whatever way he asked. Even before he spoke, I knew he was going to say, *Yes, you can. Yes, you can give me what I need for this pain without knowing anything else about me except that I'm in agony.*

But instead he asked, "You think I'm an addict, don't you?"

Sometimes, this strange, crowded room feels like a magical land. I get the sense that what the patient and I are saying to each other is not real. Sometimes the exam table seems to grow monstrous, the window's glass darkens, the walls bow inward. Sometimes, after I release a breath I don't know I am holding, I understand at what close quarters I work all day with patients. With Dan's question, the feeling of being rushed, the sense that there had only been one question hanging over the entire visit— Will you give me something for my pain?—passed. His question was an admission.

When Dan knew that *I knew* he was an addict, the spell was broken.

I have seen every kind. Some addicts are solemn; others are terrifying, and comical. I have met each kind forty times before, and they all emit a sense of neediness. At first it's a banal, impersonal neediness. I keep a restricted emotional tone while they run their lists of symptoms and complaints. Often, they are impertinent, but I don't really mind. I think the worst of each addict from the start, and then I wait for the evidence that his habit isn't so bad, it doesn't involve violence or the physical abuse of others. I wait for the part of the story that will make me think well of her, something about her that I can like as much as I dislike her addiction. It is an absurd method, but it is my way of accepting that addiction is the core of a patient's adult existence, and my job is to help him or her do something about that. Addiction intrigues me.

Some part of us believes that addiction is contagious. Children and adults are susceptible. We worry our children will catch it, and we are nothing as a country if not a giant child protection agency. I am as vigilant as the next parent. The first time my then eight-year-old son picked up his aunt's PalmPilot, he found his way to the one game loaded onto the machine, *Dope Wars.* He had to ask what dope was (as we worked through the first screens, he also asked about weed, ludes, speed, PCP, 'shrooms, and acid, although he'd heard of heroin and cocaine), and although he had no interest in keeping track of the pharmaceutical particulars, he understood immediately that the goal of this game was to make money. At eight, he had his own savings account and knew stock market basics; he figured out quickly that buying dope at a low price and selling high was strategically sound in *Dope Wars,* too. At the end of his first hour, he told me he liked the game because,

"It was easy to get really, really rich, and it was fun to shoot police." He shot them, not only out of fun, but because they were after his drugs for themselves. The game had no pictures, no moving cartoons, it was all text and yet was action packed. After you paid back the loan sharks, you had thirty days to grow your illicit bank account. You could shop for drugs all over New York, but it took valuable time to move between neighborhoods. Not only could you buy drugs, but also trench coats with larger and deeper pockets to hold your purchases, and of course, weapons. If you were lucky, you found a dead guy on the subway who carried a cache of cocaine you could rip off and then sell. You were unlucky if you were robbed at gunpoint.

The game was an education in the marketplace and at a certain level, I approved. But my son wasn't selling pork bellies—as a city kid, commodities would have been more foreign to him than heroin, and harder to describe—but drugs of abuse. I was as fascinated by the premise of *Dope Wars* as he was, but I had the grim paternal duty of explaining to him about addiction and about cocaine, heroin, and weed; I also threw in a few words against other addictive drugs he'd actually seen, alcohol and nicotine. Using my serious, moral voice, I left out all the reasons he and a million other Americans might be interested in *Dope Wars,* why in the year 2000, the PalmPilot had *this* game loaded instead of a thousand others.

Narcotics have deep roots in American culture. They entered early-nineteenth-century America through Boston traders who broke the British monopoly in opium exports from Turkey and China. Soon after the Civil War—where morphine, opium's active ingredient, was first used to relieve pain—half a million pounds of opium were arriving annually. After the war, narcotics, sold in pharmacies, were used principally by the middle class for anxiety and mood-related symptoms. Heroin, synthesized from morphine by Bayer, the company that invented aspirin, was introduced in 1896 as a cough suppressant and caught on fast. Reformers drew up tariff laws, making legal importation expensive. Trafficking began even before heroin became illegal. Today, taking Vicodin, the early twenty-first century's most popular medicinal opiate, is not a crime, but buying it without a prescription or selling it outside a pharmacy, is.

I am strangely tolerant of opiate addicts, once I get to know them. I am not exactly in favor of legalization of any currently illicit drug, but I am genuinely unhappy with jails full of Dans. Although I've been persuaded that legitimate pain sometimes requires opiates, I also know that for some people the first opiate leads to trouble. As one addict told me years ago, "If God made anything better, He kept it for himself."

Three elements are present in every story I've heard about narcotic addiction: availability, permission, and vulnerability. For the adults I see in my office, availability is never a problem. Julia was thirty-three years old, the happily married mother of young twins and owner of a successful interior decorating company; she was tall and awkwardly shy with a perfectly round face and blond bangs. She had a tiny triangular mouth touched with red lipstick. She had never tried a Vicodin until she walked into a medical center at the local mall for one of her recurring sinus infections. She had always handled the aching pain with aspirin, but now she was given antibiotics and twenty-five Vicodin. She had never even seen a Vicodin before.

"Once I took one, I realized how I felt I could get everything I needed to get done," Julia said. "I could handle stress. I was superhuman: I got things done and stayed calm, and didn't slip behind with all the work at home. It also helped with sleep."

She didn't strike me as the type who would come with an

opiate addiction looking for buprenorphine. But what is the type? A person with a particular idea of a better life? The unlucky? The monstrous? The miserable? Julia's initial Vicodin prescription might have been readily available, but the second? How did she get it? Did she experience relief of sinus pain with the first pill or was it something else—relief from the distress of infants crying? Is relief the greatest form of pleasure to an addict? Did Julia shudder a little to know she was trespassing into the forbidden? How quickly did she establish a private ritual, carried out behind closed doors, in her car, in the ladies' room, and did this privacy enable her to return to usual life pretending it hadn't occurred?

No addict starts at full speed. It isn't as if addicts try their drug once and that is it, life as they know it is over. There is a scene in *The French Connection,* where the detective, played by Gene Hackman, was kidnapped and injected with heroin by the drug dealers he's after. They were trying to show him what it was like, how good their product was. When he was released, he'd become an addict. One dose and he was hooked. In real life, this never happens. But it is a common misconception. A person becomes an addict after weeks or months of regular use, escalating out-of-control, desperate, problematic use, despite the addict talking her- or himself into thinking things are okay. You can talk yourself into anything if you repeat it enough.

Opiate addiction doesn't happen to everyone who takes a Vicodin. But there are some people who, like Julia, can't leave behind the new feeling Vicodin provides.

Julia used Vicodin (they look like, but are a little larger than, aspirin) twice a day as prescribed for two weeks, along with her sinus infection–clearing antibiotics, but when the infection was resolved and the sinus pain went away, she held on to the remaining Vicodin. At first, she used her leftover pills only on stressful days at home when her husband was out of town. Then she tried one or two at special events, at weddings and funerals; then for celebrations or injuries; then after an exceptional meal. She asked for Vicodin with her next sinus infection. Later, months later, when she'd gotten herself another prescription, she gave herself permission to take one when she was happy or bored, depressed, anxious, or angry. One of those feelings always seemed to be available around the time she was going to use, and using became a daily occurrence.

She made certain rules as the months went on—never extra doses beyond what she really needed during the workweek, one extra pill to make it through an afternoon when a relative visited—but the rules kept changing. When Julia read the side effect profile that came from the pharmacy, she thought: This pill isn't obviously dangerous, not like booze or cigarettes. Vicodin had acetaminophen in it, which in excess could cause liver problems, but drinking and smoking ruined your body, destroyed blood and tissue.

When Julia first came to see me, she said, "My husband knew I wasn't sleeping well, but he didn't know the half of it. I was embarrassed and didn't want to admit my problem. When did I become so sneaky? I said to myself, *Taper off the Vicodin.* I thought I could get through it. But physically, I felt so bad trying to stop. I'd give up after only a day. I kept telling myself, *I'll try again tomorrow.* That's when I realized I had a drug problem, and I didn't know how to get myself out of it. I thought getting drug treatment meant going away to rehab like they do on TV, and there was no way I could do that with two little girls at home. So I figured I was doomed until I read about buprenorphine."

There is no single moment when a person becomes addicted. It is slow, gradual, insidious. Addicts deny addiction for as long as possible, and finally accept it numbly. Julia admitted she'd had a blind spot about what she was doing. Vicodin had become a new requirement in her life—and so did sneaking pills in and out of her drawers and her pocketbooks.

If we believe that genes dictate our fates, we accept that every addict has a special vulnerability. This was how Lucy Fields viewed herself: her susceptibility was just waiting to be exposed. It erupted as soon as she started drugs as an adolescent. But the risk of addiction can be latent into one's thirties or forties (as in Julia's case). We might not express this vulnerability as teenagers, but instead it can come out under the right conditions—for instance, the stress of having two children under four years old.

We live in an era of brain science and are told that behaviors such as addiction come about because of an interaction between susceptibility and precipitant, between our genetic makeup and our environment. If an addict doesn't have a strong family history of alcoholism or other substance use, his addiction might be a consequence of trauma. Culturally, we sense that addicts are injured people. It really doesn't matter what kind of trauma it is. A violent parent, the death of a beloved relative, abandonment, too little love, sexual abuse, the overwhelming stress of war—any of these might create a microscopic biological injury that is transiently relieved by drugs like Vicodin. But those who do not believe that addiction is the result of some genetic fate might think that Julia's or Lucy's behavior was the result of a personal failing—a moral or spiritual weakness. Since every reasonable American believes it is virtuous to control one's behavior, the addicted men and women who come to my office simply didn't want to deny themselves. Their fervor was of the wrong kind. They wanted to live a certain way, never mind the consequences. They *willed* their opiate use, went looking for it, perhaps abetted by life context, surroundings, a few influential people who also used.

Tom was a funeral director who was given a prescription for

Percocet after a bicycle accident left him with neck pain. Percocet gave him a buzz. But he would be the first to tell you that Percocet made his mind become pleasantly numb, and he was very open to being deadened in those months after his divorce. Opiates do not affect everyone in the same way—Tom felt anesthetized, Julia physically energized and dangerously alive—but most people feel nothing more than pain relief, a little nausea, a little dizzy; this last group never becomes addicted.

By the time Julia sought care, she didn't feel "superhuman"; she felt like a disappointment. Shame was easy to detect—it didn't look like pain or fatigue. It resembled a foot caught in a trap. She was deeply humiliated that she had ever begun taking pills. She had a lot to save in her day-to-day life; she wanted to get back to the way things were. Julia wanted to feel less nervous, but entering my office made her extremely anxious. Using Vicodin allowed her to have certain feelings and to avoid others. It was a way of shifting focus, of deflecting or skipping past self-awareness, of finding ease or courage or energy.

Every addict can come up with reasons to take the next pill. This comes easily because they are being driven by a deep pull, a yearning for the next, that eventually becomes a strong crippling need. As Julia admitted at her first visit, "I didn't feel addicted. I just wanted more." But she had moved from dependent to addicted when she lied to her husband, when she used extra pills to get through the stress of a family weekend.

Once she was using every six or eight hours, she no longer required reasons to use, she was just trying to avoid the sickness of opiate withdrawal. Physically dependent, Julia wasn't looking forward to the next pill with enthusiasm. On a Vicodin schedule, she never quite felt settled, except for a thin slice of time around dosing, when the drug entered her bloodstream and brain. She couldn't function without it, couldn't come close to being who she imagined she was without it. She kept doing it even as Vicodin was ruining the things she cared about.

For better or worse, people tell me remarkable things. Surprisingly, this is not only true of addicts, and not only true in my office. Within minutes, strangers—at a gym class, on a plane, in the grocery line—talk to me. They tell me their sexual adventures, ethical transgressions, financial nightmares. I've tried to understand why they speak so openly; perhaps it's because I've never had trouble giving someone my full attention. And the less I have in common with them, the easier it is for me to listen. In my office, I stress informality and spontaneity and the idea that patients are leaving me soon, so if they have something important to say, they might as well put it out there. Patients speak about things they can't believe they've done; they recollect and brood. If a new patient doesn't touch upon something embarrassing or previously unacknowledged, I'm disappointed.

It's difficult to be mad at an elderly emphysema patient who admits she has been using some of her sister's sleeping pills, or at the heart failure patient who overdoses every Sunday night on Chinese food. These patients disappoint, annoy, even frustrate me, but they don't make me angry. But with addicts like Dan, who push me to respond, who show malice, I never feel badly when I angrily offer them no satisfaction.

Dan finally sat in the chair with a big show of effort, as if he had just done me a favor. I proposed writing him a prescription for ten Percocet and making an appointment for Monday so we might talk more about what was actually going on here. It was a deal, a compromise. Ten pills would do him no harm and might stop him from visiting an emergency room that night with another manufactured complaint.

"Ten? Only ten?" He was outraged. He was convinced that I was discriminating against him. Usually my white coat stopped people from being rude, but not Dan. "How's that going to help? I'm in pain."

As he leaped up and threw open the door, I knew I would not see him again. I knew he was resourceful and could find Percocet elsewhere.

I'd made him a fair proposition I thought—but as I drove home, I wondered what had gone wrong and was only able to determine that we had altogether different agendas. There was no way we could come up with a plan that would suit us both.

There was a good chance that Dan had been manipulative and difficult long before he ever tried Percocet. I try to be polite and cordial with patients, but it isn't always possible. Sometimes I have bad days—for example, when my basement flooded for the third time in the spring, when my left knee's tendonitis flared. But I also have to remind myself not to give in to a kind of superior tone. Superiority is a weapon. Superiority leads me to a TV-drama-shaped inclination to turn each medical visit into a moral lesson, and the more intense I am in my demands with addicts, the more strained and exasperated, the less successful I am in getting them to change.

Most days, I sympathize and listen and say the things doctors are supposed to say, but inside, I am shaking my head at the wreckage and obsession. Patients who are addicts know they've had a problem for months or even years. They know this is why a child was taken away by DCYF, why they've lost their job and house. In private, they make the connection between misery and drugs, even as they try to maintain appearances.

Etymologically, addiction means surrender. To what? Surrender to a certain kind of pleasure: a relief from human contact, a relief from one's own thoughts and company. Getting high is to get rid of one's self; it is sending the self away. To be high is to have known something once, but to have forgotten it. Opiates bring pleasure, and people take pleasure where they can find it, and when they are addicted, pleasure can't be refused, deferred, denied.

We presume that too much of any pleasure-giving substance will inevitably result in a crash. After all, the addict is, by definition, out of control.

If Julia, Tom, or Lucy had come in to discuss high blood pressure and admitted incidentally to using narcotics *only occasionally*, for pleasure, what would I have told them other than the obvious: that they had chosen enjoyments that were illegal? Would I have downplayed this pleasure if they downplayed the possible danger of becoming hooked? Why shouldn't they find enjoyment in their own ways? Two Vicodin rather than two gin and tonics? Even used heavily, opiates rarely disturb memory or rationality. However, my sense is that over time opiates have a considerable effect on judgment and emotions, but in a less overt and acute way than alcohol, which more obviously affects reactions, balance, and behavior.

I had one patient, Monica, who used heroin only on weekends, who never became addicted, whose life was not in shambles. A striking woman with dyed black hair and a red anvil necklace, she came to see me for her asthma. Monica spoke of her relationship with heroin as a love affair. Heroin energized her, made her feel at her peak physically, helped her focus. She didn't "need" heroin, and she thought of those whose drug use was uncontrollable as weak. She didn't accept the equivalence of opiate use and addiction. Her definition of an addict was someone who allowed opiates to structure her calendar and mood, who acted surprised when she shouldn't have been that some part of life—family, finances—was ruined by drugs. For Monica, who had a fine income as the manager of jewelry store, heroin was a luxury; she didn't need it any more than she needed a new dress, and she knew it was laughable to imply that one could have a dress addiction. Addiction was a choice, a mentality, but not a disease.

Heroin satisfied Monica, took care of her in full; it was not difficult for her to describe its terrific lure. An opera lover, she described the experience of getting high as like entering an ingeniously designed auditorium where she had been given an excellent seat. It was a vast empty space that somehow afforded an intimacy with the performance; she was in the audience but was also the performer, the soloist. And what a strange, hybrid performance: grippingly worldly and cosmopolitan, but sung silently, heroin was an absence that reverberated through her body. The first fifteen minutes of every dose were consistently better than any other performance in her life, incomparable, and she could get a ticket whenever she wanted.

Monica was sure of who she was and she was reluctant to change (even though we discussed the plausible relationship of her asthma to her heroin inhalation), yet she kept coming to see me. When I asked what it would take to make her quit, she was neither perfunctory nor evasive. She laughed. "I am completely unwilling to give up heroin."

My twenty years of practice have taught me that Monica is the exception—patients who take narcotics for pleasure have a hard time limiting themselves. It is extremely rare to find a patient who can calibrate the exact amount needed for pleasure without slipping into dependence. If Vicodin can provide an infinite supply of pleasure, it is wildly frustrating for some people not to take full advantage; these are the ones who make it to my office. For those who use only occasionally, the future is always a test.

Lucy Fields had failed the test. Near the end of her first visit, she said to me, "By the time people are my age, they're married and have children. They've had friends for a long time. I haven't seen anyone from college or high school in ten years. I haven't really been in the business of making friends. I have no family living in this state, no savings, no job, only a boyfriend who's an addict, too." When addicts beginning treatment speak of "recovery," they are only hoping to become drug free.

Perhaps addicts interest me in the way some people are interested in celebrities. Like addicts, celebrities' ambitions are the manifestation of private desires: urgent, insistent, simple. I admire vehement passions. I love the plays of Shakespeare. I applaud emotion that often trumps reason, and I don't presume that people always act in their best interest. I hear it every day in my office from patients with coronary artery disease and diabetes and rheumatoid arthritis: I planned on saving for a new winter coat, but I spent my entire paycheck on a new car; I planned to take the new medication you prescribed, but I got scared; I was planning to be faithful to my husband, but I found myself having sex with another man; I was planning to give up Vicodin, but I couldn't resist one more pill. In the moment, temptations can arise that trip our plans. Although I know that enthusiasm could be pathological, addiction is what I expect passion to be—when it gets hold of you, it is not gentle or fair.

Unlike Julia, Lucy didn't want the past back; unlike Monica, she wanted the future to be different. For ten years, using Vicodin daily, she had lost track of time; wanting to quit was a signal that she was again aware of time passing. "What do you want your life to be like in a year?" I asked Lucy at our first visit.

"Simple basic things I'd be satisfied with," she said. "My own place to live. Productive work. I still don't know what happened to me."

"Why do want to go to South Carolina?" I'd asked.

"Because now that we've discussed it, my mother would be miserable if I didn't. I feel obligated. I've never visited their place since they bought it five years ago.

"Plus my father bought a turntable. A turntable for old vinyl records. I know that sounds funny, but they're coming back into fashion. He has hundreds of records that I remember him playing when I was young, and I'd like to hear them again."

Her rich, sudden, dense laugh made her presence nervous and exciting. Was Lucy truly interested in quitting Vicodin? I had no idea.

CHAPTER 3

Monday, April 21

I wasn't at all sure that Lucy Fields would return. Drug users make promises they don't keep. They try and they fail. That's how it works. They just can't do it sometimes.

I've never believed the popular saying that addicts seek care only once they "hit bottom." Addicts don't come in at the bottom, but when the future somehow looks worse than where they were now. Lucy's situation sounded as if it might get worse—newly jobless, growing problems with boyfriend.

I had plans for Lucy, but they may not have been the same ones she had for herself. It had only been five days since her first visit, but I was beginning to think she saw no role for me in her future. I had a medication to offer, but I couldn't repair her. I could offer balance, I could make her alert to what was good in the world, but I couldn't take away her angers and disappointments and sadness. She would have to leave those aside for now.

After our session, she likely went straight home to her Vicodin. It is easier to continue opiates than to quit. Many addicts, looking to quit, tell themselves they are only taking a break. They refuse to think: I will *never* use again. That would be too extreme.

What Lucy likely knew was that the beginning of buprenorphine treatment would be the worst because it involved going through a Vicodin hiatus (and the start of opiate withdrawal) before receiving the first dose of medication. Even when addicts are certain that it is better to be free of Vicodin, heroin, or OxyContin, they waver. When they look back over any year, the only periods that stand out are those when they'd run out and been "drug sick," in withdrawal. Using three or four times every day makes for routine, a two-dimensional, directed life—I'm using now, I know when I will need to use again.

This morning, Lucy entered my office wobbly, uncomfortable, in a sweat. Many addicts stay up late, take their last dose, and awake starting to withdraw and crave opiates. Morning is the worst time of day for most addicts, and I had asked Lucy to come when she was many hours into withdrawal. Could any opiate-dependent person quit cold turkey without a day of drug sickness? I have heard of such people, and maybe they are somewhere out there, but I have never met one.

Tall and thin, Lucy moved heavily, slowly, like a song decelerating toward its final bars. Her skin was dull gray and blotchy, her eyes a morose blue. She seemed indifferent to the way she looked. She had none of the vivaciousness of the first visit when she spoke openly, as if she'd been holding in and concentrating her thoughts for a decade. All that mattered now was that her last

Vicodin was fourteen hours before, at 6:00 P.M. As every mor
after midnight had arrived, and the Vicodin continued to slip ot
the opiate receptors in her brain, she knew she would not be able
to continue without some respite. Her desire to use was so powerful her head was ready to burst.

"I'm back," she said, glancing at me, blinking, her chin jerking
and then looking away. Her face was vacant, distancing herself
from the pain. She went to her chair, looking toward the door or
floor, or if toward me, over my head.

"I'm glad," I answered.

Vicodin produces almost no withdrawal symptoms until it has
been used for at least two weeks. But as one uses more and more,
withdrawal starts to creep up on the person after even a half day
off. For some opiate users, the first indication that they have a
problem is when they notice the signs of withdrawal; usually they
stop before things get worse. But those who come to my buprenorphine program have taken a different path; they have dealt
with withdrawal by using more opiates.

At most medical visits, the patient arrives with the question:
What's wrong with me? The question comes in the form of a
symptom I might identify. Why can't I catch my breath walking
uphill, what is this bump behind my ear, why are my feet swollen? Lucy arrived knowing exactly what was wrong—she knew
better than I would ever know—because she had produced the
symptoms herself. She had spent her entire addiction avoiding
these feelings, and knowing exactly how to relieve them. It is
called a "fix," after all, because those pills fix you right up, repair
you, when withdrawal begins.

For Lucy, these first hours were a struggle, a negative ecstasy.
When she took Vicodin, it reached not only her brain, but also
her fingers and legs. Now all of those places hurt. There was no

legs, just pain. Some addicts believe that they get pain, not in spite of it. But not Lucy. Every bodily distilled, every movement too self-aware. To be in s to experience a combination of urgent frustration and hyped-up concentration.

Sobriety would not come easily, and it was not easy to watch a person assimilate the inrush of agony. A person in pain can't stand to stay in her own body, but there was no escape. Lucy was waiting to feel better amid an overwhelming sense of hopeless grief. I knew when I saw her she had begun a slow, steady pace, a jog, toward a new equilibrium, but she had none of the eagerness of a woman who saw a maximum of a future for herself.

Lucy was giving up something that would leave her feeling that she was less than the woman she had been for ten years. Losing her Vicodin felt like an amputation, a disfigurement. Even though I was giving her a new drug to replace the old one, it wouldn't be the same. Buprenorphine would disperse itself in her body slowly and steadily and wouldn't get her high (not that Vicodin did either anymore, although it still had that memory attached). And I was asking her to use it on my schedule, not her own. She knew she would need to take buprenorphine only once a day and that she would go to the pharmacy to buy it, rather than depending on her boyfriend for a supply.

"I can't believe you sent me out last Wednesday and said to come back in five days," she chided me. "I was expecting to start your medication then, you know. When you said, basically, that I had to use Vicodin for five more days, or until yesterday, I couldn't believe it. I know you didn't *tell* me to keep using, but you knew I would, you knew I had to." She directed her gaze at my knees.

She was telling me I had already let her down—that I had

not done enough. And yet I knew I had said enough of the right things for her to come back today having put herself in pain.

"It was a matter of scheduling and making sure you were in withdrawal. I know you're going through the worst part," I said.

Opiate withdrawal arrives in predictable stages, each signaling greater loss of control of one's body. Early on, there is yawning and piloerection (goose bumps), nose-dripping and eye-watering and a general achiness. The insidious attack on the body has begun. If not interrupted, it will lead to vomiting and diarrhea, chills and sweats. The mind sends word to the body that it has been hit, and that blow will soon transmit to every muscle, organ, limb.

Cocaine wears off quickly but not the opiates. Cocaine's lift lasts ten minutes and creates the urgent desire to use more. But after the cocaine is gone, the body forgets it, leaving behind a rancid irritability. Taking an opiate is like eating a big meal; afterward you are satisfied, sleepy, full, warm next to a fire, and that feeling doesn't wear off for hours. But when it does, it is as if you are starving, each cold cell is hungry, and you haven't eaten in days. (Most opiate addicts are nostalgic for the first high they've ever had; they still mourn the loss of that feeling, which was somehow better than any other.)

"I didn't know if I'd make it back today."

"But you did."

Below each of her cheekbones was the smoothed, healed acne craters that must have reminded her every day of a difficult adolescence. She wasn't wearing any makeup, and that made her look older than I remembered. The lack of makeup was evidence that any semblance of self-care had been discarded, but also, metaphorically, that she was facing this withdrawal period uncovered.

There is endless anxiety available to the addict, but the primal anxiety of withdrawal, a heavy feeling, is different. Many addicts know the anxiety of getting arrested, losing a job, getting discovered by a spouse or lover. Withdrawal anxiety is physical: every cell ready to mutiny; the arrival of a graveyard stink of sweat; a feeling of impossibility. In the middle of the night, Lucy must have been thinking: If I use Vicodin now, I will be rewarding myself, but also letting myself down. He will not take me in the program. She did not have to tell me any of this. Instead, she pressed her knees together and tightened her lips.

"Yesterday, I cleaned out my stash so I wouldn't have any to take when it started to get bad," she said. In the middle of the night, she had to decide whether to battle or walk away. By 4:00 A.M., the manic agitation and moodiness had probably proceeded to delusional thinking and obsessional fantasy: *I know I left a Vicodin around here somewhere. Where is it?* Hadn't she kept one in the house in case she couldn't stand these feelings a minute longer? Or had she truly cleared her medicine cabinet and her sock drawer and her pocketbook so that she wouldn't have an easy source nearby?

She wanted to flee now. I imagined her driving to the bay. Somehow the beach would suit her this morning. She could swim in the icy water. She stiffened, trembled, grew numb. Her mouth went dry, her throat tightened. Her mind had flown out of her body. The line between thinking and saying became blurred: *Did I say that or just think it?* She was confused. The last hours had been like dying in the darkness of her room, and if she wasn't dying, she wanted to kill herself.

When she hit the twelfth hour after her last pill, she couldn't have imagined feeling worse. This, the sixteenth hour, was worse. Her stomach was likely ruined beyond salvage. She twisted and pulled her knees up. It was terrible to watch. Abdominal cramping had begun in inevitable waves. No longer was she thinking, *Look at me, I'm flying*. It was, *Look at me, I'm falling*. But no one dies from narcotic withdrawal as one does from opiate overdose. I've heard opiate addicts say, "I need my heroin like a diabetic needs his insulin," but that isn't a physiologically accurate analogy. You don't die without narcotics. There is no risk of dying from stopping Vicodin, alone in your room at night.

Withdrawal, with its ties to terror and shame, inspires a powerful desire to hide. This is why nearly half of the addicts I meet at a first visit never return. But when they do come back for a second visit, it is still a surprise to me. For those who return, the fear of failure is great—why start what can't be sustained?—but an eagerness to try is greater.

Every addict tries to be brave and strong as his or her symptoms set in. The burden of this withdrawal visit is what invests the addict with bravery, a kind of nobility I admire. How do addicts give themselves courage? They grab hold of their own wrists. They take out combs and brush madly. They sit on their hands. Lucy, for the second time, sat on her legs, pinning herself to the chair. Lucy was not a moaner, a complainer. She didn't fuss.

Withdrawal is a necessary condition for success with buprenorphine. At ten in the morning in my office, Lucy was sick and scared and had come in alone.

"Well, here I am, in pain, as you probably expected. Now where are we?" she asked. She still hadn't looked up. She rubbed her palms together to dampen her impatience. She was irritable; her body was like a hive.

Now where are we? Meaning: I've done what you asked, now what will you do for me?

Patients expect me to look them in the eyes. If I don't, they think something is wrong with me. Lucy had avoided my eyes the first visit, and she was looking away again today. Out of respect, I managed to look attentively at either side of her face, trying not to catch her glance until she looked for mine. Not looking her in the eye, I thought, might make her feel there was not quite so much loaded against her.

"I'll need to do a brief physical exam and then we can get you some buprenorphine," I said.

To have a patient leave my office without a check of her blood pressure, without listening to her lungs, seemed negligent. As an internist, it is what I do for every other patient under my care. When a patient enters my office, I typically take a medical history and move on to an examination. The cardiac patient's exam focuses on the heart and lungs, and legs, where fluid pools. The examination of the cancer patient is often a search for lymph nodes and bony tenderness. With the arthritis patient, I study every joint, toe to shoulder.

I would look at exactly the same things on Lucy as I did on every patient. I had to examine her because it is what I am trained to do, and because one reason addicts come to internists is to have a doctor who can manage general medical problems as well as addiction. The bodies of drug users reveal particular bits of information. I would spend a little longer looking at certain parts of Lucy. Drug injectors have scars on their arms where veins have collapsed, or skin infections where needles have left bacteria behind, and a careful look at her arms would confirm that Lucy only used pills. Drug sniffers sometimes have bleeding noses. Opiates shrink one's pupils to pinpoints. Addicts can lie about how much they use and where they use, and with whom, but if their pupils are pinned, they can't lie about being high. If Lucy was infected with one of the hepatitis viruses, she might have an enlarged liver, which I could detect by placing my hands below the edge of her ribs on her right.

"Whatever you have to do," Lucy said. I am always a little surprised by the yielding of serious, intelligent people. In this room, I can ask things of people I can ask nowhere else.

I rose and walked over to the green examining table, which is formed on a mild slope and comes in three sections with a hanging but liftable extension piece at one end for people with long legs. There is a small airline-ish pillow to put under the head or knees. I took a gown from one of the table's drawers. This half of my office, closer to the window, where the examining table stands, felt temporary, anonymous, easily wiped down. The smell was almost too clean, as if disease was far away and not in the person in front of me.

"If you could put this on," I said, handing over the crimson material, "and just leave on your underwear. I'll be back in a minute."

I excused myself from the room.

Women always cover as much as possible. Some women refuse to see male doctors after bad experiences, and this seems understandable to me. But plenty of women are unbothered by the kind of touching they expect from any doctor. Probing, poking fingers are uncomfortable no matter what gender they are attached to. Any woman who visits a male doctor expects cordiality and the appropriate hesitancies and requests (the heart, on the left side of the chest, is always a tricky place to reach, the gown lowered, the stethoscope positioned) and makes this clear through the alertness of her eyes; any tension the doctor experiences is his problem.

When I returned, Lucy was wearing the magenta dressing gown I'd left her. She sat, socks on, bare legs dangling, at the edge of the table. She was thin, a little slouched. Her slenderness made me wonder if she could finish an entire grilled cheese. She was looking off to the side as if trying to think of something. She sat with her hands on her bare knees like a tired hostess after a long party. To be examined, to be naked even under a gown, strips us down to our defenseless essence, our original helpless state; maybe she was thinking of this.

Every examination has a formal pattern, even if it is abbreviated as it was with Lucy. I tried not to proceed by intuition but by order. I couldn't afford to get tired or forgetful. The choreography was rehearsed and minimal—blood pressure, eyes, mouth, lungs, chest, legs, arms—but hardly dull. Touching a stranger's body always makes the examiner feel intensely alive, awake. But I could never let on that I was feeling this at all.

Doctors and patients have a pact. The patient makes herself free to be touched, but how and where the doctor lays his hand will never be mentioned between them or, if done sensitively and correctly, to anyone else. It is possible for both parties to be unembarrassed, but it is difficult not to avert the eyes.

Every patient feels in danger when being touched by a doctor. He or she has a lingering suspicion: What can he tell by touching me? The patient thinks about what might be discovered not only *in* me or *on* me, but *about* me? What is below the surface, what set of problems? The examination makes connections between the invisible and the visible world, and the doctor's job is to look for what is identifiably wrong; he is searching for the difficult and dangerous. Patients are comforted only when the exam is over and an all-clear sign has been given.

Lucy sat grimly—sad, determined, worn-out, unbowed. I knew this was very difficult for her. I could tell she didn't like being looked at. To examine someone who has submitted only because she can't refuse insults them and demeans me.

I flashed a light in her eyes and in her open mouth. Her teeth were perfect, ticker-tape white, with a single filling in the back. The state of her teeth was a sign of middle-class upbringing. Bad teeth are most often a sign of poverty (the last item on a to-do list), but also of madness or despair. The public's association of addiction with poverty is part of what makes the addict culturally contemptible, but more than a lack of cash, a patient's ruined mouth signals a general lack of self-care.

Lucy didn't look. She couldn't. She lay back. Her stomach made airy, high-pitched sounds. The table was narrow enough that she would fall off if she did not lie still, so she kept her arms in close, a stiff position. She fixed her eyes on the ceiling before she closed them, feigning sleep, the posture of the enchanted princess. She tried to make powerlessness into ease. There was a pointlessness to moving or complaining. She listened for her own shallow breathing and her heart beating. Looking closely at someone who is horizontal is always intimate. She had to wait until I was finished, that's all. And hope that she could begin her treatment soon.

I prefer not to speak during an examination; my thoughts are in my fingers. Some patients talk during the entire examination in order to distract themselves from the ticklishness, the fear, the closeness. I concentrate more fully if they are quiet. The trick is to move over another's body without any trace of emotion.

I moved quickly, keeping a mental checklist of the few potential irregularities I was looking for. It was unlikely I would find anything that would prevent me from prescribing buprenorphine. I lifted or parted only those sections of her gown that I needed to and maneuvered a second gown I'd taken from the drawer to conceal her unnecessarily uncovered areas. When she opened her eyes, I tapped on her echoic and slightly tender belly. She sunk into the table the way a boxer used the ropes to help absorb an opponent's blows.

The skin of her arms and hands was like the sheet on a bed you've left, crumpled, pale, and dusky. She was dehydrated. She probably hadn't had much to drink after the inevitable nausea set in. As with all my patients, I was careful to look once, and if I did again, I risked causing alarm. Sometimes it was an effort to be casual. Sometimes I had to pretend I'd noticed nothing. I meant for my gaze to give nothing away until I was finished and we could speak later, after she had dressed, in our roles of doctor and patient, rather than undressed woman and white-coated man.

Every few moments, I glanced at Lucy's face. I needed the visual testimony of pain. Agony rested in her body, but her pain was also psychic. Maybe she was saving her energy. But I also thought that she was displaying her newfound strength for me, and for herself. Addiction is a feeling of wanting something, and she was showing me how little she wanted or needed this morning.

Her smell was mineral, like a towel not fully dried. I breathed on the bell of my stethoscope to warm it. I pressed it against her and realized I was listening hard to avoid looking at her chest; opening her eyes was a way of telling me to move on. She sat up and I listened again to her heart. I looked into her nostrils and pressed on her sinuses. The tip of her nose was cold.

Touching her—the resistance of her muscles, the tension of her forehead's skin, the angles of her wrists, the movements of her toes—gave some sense of her suspicions, sadness, and readiness to collapse, and also of how she took approval, what calmed and encouraged her. Every working body is the same, but every body holds determination and frustration and worry and weakness differently.

"I hate being touched," she said when the exam was over. As she sat up, I saw that her body's impression had been sweated into the white butcher paper on the exam table. "I don't like dentists. Sitting in a chair and having someone stand over me. I hate it. Dentists, doctors, hairdressers. I don't like it when anyone tries to touch me." She sat at the end of my table, heavy armed and light-headed. She groaned and shuddered. Her neck was stiff, her fists balled. The sweat on her back was like cold rain.

I washed my hands in the silver sink, used the paper towel dispenser above it. As soon as an examination is over, the patient wants to hear what I'd found and be gone. The primary value of a physical exam in someone young and healthy is reassurance. Lucy could be eased in only one way. She wanted her medication. Withdrawal had created an uneasy, deep discomfort, and she wanted it to disappear. She wanted buprenorphine not as a "cure" but as an unglamorous, unthrilling way of regaining the life that had been taken away.

"Your exam is completely normal," I said. "I'm going to step out so that you can get dressed, and then we'll get you some relief."

In the hall, I had a little time. I eased into the conference room two doors down to cadge a muffin and spent a few minutes reading the headlines about the war in Iraq, which set me thinking about and fearing for my talented and brave nephews, completing college and preparing to enlist—Marines Officer Training School, Quantico. I also wondered about my colleague Mark, a flight surgeon in the Reserve, called up a month before, and tried to remember, yet again, his wife's name and whether he had four or five kids. I eavesdropped in on the old argument between nursing assistants about who last had the keys to the copy machine room, and about food stored in the staff refrigerator. Then I stretched my legs by walking the length of our office space toward the file room, passing the Portuguese cleaning duo who leaned toward the music coming from a radio tucked in a bucket of rags at the end of the hall.

Over the years I've heard stories of addicts who got themselves off opiates by locking themselves in a room (Miles Davis famously isolated himself in his parents' farmhouse), but this is rare. They tried to cure their suffering with more suffering. If the ordeal was profound, they might remember it aversively so they would never use opiates again. But it is extremely difficult to go cold turkey and "cure" oneself. The sickness Lucy Fields was now experiencing would be intense for forty-eight hours but would continue for five to eight days. Day by day her body would grow increasingly raw and twitchy, as if she were covered in dry ice, that slow burn. Twelve or sixteen hours might be tolerable, but eight days was too long for most addicts to go it alone. No doctor suggests this harsh, medically unsupervised treatment; we don't like to hurt people, to stand by (figuratively) withholding help as they suffer. Many opiate addicts seek a weeklong supervised withdrawal, commonly known as "detox." Detoxification is a scheduled tapering off of the opiate, combined with enough sleeping medications to knock one out for the worst of it. But detox is hardly a cure; after detox, fewer than 5 percent of addicts stay off their drug permanently; most relapse soon after leaving. The psyche cannot be taken apart and reassembled in a week.

Lucy and I had reviewed the options to treat her opiate dependence during her first visit. The buprenorphine would reverse the withdrawal symptoms by substituting for Vicodin. But more than one doctor, more than one former patient, more than one spouse of a patient, has told me that replacing Vicodin (or heroin or OxyContin) with buprenorphine is simply exchanging one opiate for another. Buprenorphine is an opiate, too, after all, albeit one that produces no euphoria. I was complicit, a narcotic dealer in a white coat. Why don't I let an addict cut free from substances altogether?

I often have to justify my "program" in a world where it is not clear what addicts suffer from, whether addiction is part of one's basic character structure (which would not be expected to be particularly malleable) or an acute condition that can be treated. Every opinion about what should be done to help addicts is controversial, whereas the optimal treatment of asthma is a matter of clinical nuance, not ideology. Buprenorphine treatment in my program is a long-term commitment; I recommend that patients who start buprenorphine stay on it for months before making a decision about coming off it.

The reason I suggested buprenorphine for Lucy was the same one I offer all opiate addicts: although buprenorphine would continue her physical dependence on opiates, it had another binding force—it bound her to me. Dependent on me for a prescription, Lucy would visit me regularly, and in this way I might be able to help her change a life she had been unsuccessful at changing on her own. There had to be someone who knew her secrets, someone who knew her history, and someone she depended on who was benign, goodwilled, and would have a reasonable response to her behaviors. If I believed that opiate-dependent patients could change on their own, I would hand over the magic pills and send them on their way. But I believe patients need someone. I am the emblem of the rules and structure that is needed to break their habit. I, my program, am not free and easy.

Lucy would be making a commitment not only to me, but to arranging her day differently, to keeping away from certain people and places. She would take buprenorphine and stay away from Vicodin, and when she came to see me, I would ask her to be self-absorbed, which might allow, if all went well, for the possibility of insight and behavior change. With each patient I believe the right word or gesture could spark something good in them. I believe that as a doctor I could affect life's small events, and what is wrong with that?

Just before I was about to return to Lucy's room, a nursing assistant stopped me in the hall and told me I had an urgent phone call. I had picked up the phone and a woman's voice said, "My name is Cindy." She was weeping. "You saw my husband, Dan, on Friday. I know there are rules about talking to me about him. I work with adolescents and I know about those laws. . . .

"Don't hang up," she begged.

I was shocked that Dan had a wife. Now that I was on the phone, I couldn't hang up. She could barely speak through her crying.

"There are privacy laws regarding speaking about anyone I see here," I said, careful not to admit that I even knew her husband. I tried not to say it coldly, but it came out that way. He had not said anything about his family.

"I know he was supposed to see you this morning."

He wasn't; we had no second appointment scheduled. I didn't correct her; I couldn't. I was surprised she knew he had visited my office at all.

"He's not here now," she continued, sniffling. "He went into detox. I just learned about his drug use this weekend. I knew he had an addictive personality, but I never thought we'd come to this. He emptied our bank accounts; that's how I found out. We have no money left in our savings. He took it all. He took advances on our credit cards, $10,000 and $5,000. I don't know what we're going to do. He told me he went to see you this morning and you weren't there, so he took himself to a detox program over at the hospital."

I'd been in the office all morning. One of the nursing assistants would have told me if he'd walked in. Another lie.

"I can't leave him. What would he do? I hate his parents. They've never helped him. They're awful people. I don't know what to do. We have two children. I'm all he has. When he gets out of detox in three or four days, he wants to come back to see you, he told me. He told them at detox that you were his doctor."

"He should make an appointment if he's been seen here and wants to return," I said carefully.

"Thank you. Thank you so much. He really needs help."

"You're welcome to come, too," I said softly. "It's often helpful if patients bring in the people who care about them."

I believe this is true for any patient with any condition. When patients bring in family and friends, I can get a better sense of what their lives are like outside this office. I can identify an ally who might assist me. I will have a witness, someone who can confirm my instructions, corroborate what I say. The more help patients get at home, the less uncertain and astray they feel. Addicts trying to quit are always in need of consolation. But so are their families.

"You should get some help for yourself."

After I hung up, I thought about how glad I was that Lucy had returned, and how talking to an addict was like talking to a friend who was in love with the wrong person. Vicodin whispers to its lover, "You know how I make you feel. *He* doesn't." Can you talk a person out of the wild gamble of being in love? Sometimes there is no stopping them.

I reentered the exam room where Lucy was sitting in her chair hugging her legs.

"Tell me how you are."

"I feel like shit, that's how I am," she said from a bottomless supply of indignation. Her face had a fine film of sweat, and she sat very still, as if she did not want to unsettle her stomach or head.

She could not think of another word to say. She wanted me to leave her in peace. She had spent her life concealed; right now perhaps I should let her be. I reached into my coat pocket for my pad. I wrote her name and the date across the top line of a prescription. It was for six two-milligram buprenorphine tablets, enough for today only. No refills.

"You take the elevator back down to the ground floor. You follow the signs over to the hospital pharmacy. It's about a five-minute walk. You hand them this prescription. I will call over there so they know you're coming. You bring the bottle with the six pills back to me. Don't use any of the pills before you get here. Wait in the waiting area and I'll come find you. Then I'll tell you what to do next."

I don't keep buprenorphine in my office. I could put it in a safe with a combination lock and keep a few pills in it, but I don't want an addict to ever think I have anything in my room worth stealing. I stood and led Lucy to the door, stepping into the hall to watch her leave.

The walk to the pharmacy gave her a chance to run away. It gave her the time to go a little deeper into withdrawal. It gave her time to think again about the deal we were making, the quiet agreement that any struggle between us was over, that whatever came next was already decided.

Emanating from the rooms on this hallway is the clammy aroma of fear. We work in eight-by-twelve boxes of dread up and down the corridor. In each is a different scale of upset: some monstrous, some a tiny tug of anxiety. Doctors are bound together by a collective responsibility to a community of worriers, men and women unsure of what comes next. Each patient in each room takes slow deep breaths and worries that at any moment he or she might receive news that would change them forever. Each steps into his or her doctor's room thinking: *All may not be well, but he will deliver the news and try to set things right.*

I returned to my desk and wondered again what Lucy's parents knew about all this. How suspicious were they about their daughter's life? I was sure she must have shown up sleeping but awake at family events. Did they really not ask what was going on? And if they didn't, did it mean they didn't love her, didn't care? What did they notice, recognize, acknowledge? Had they been too solicitous over the years? Was self-destruction Lucy Fields's means of communication?

I heard a knock on my door.

"Here they are," Lucy said, handing over a small white bag, stapled closed with a typed medication label. She had obviously slipped through the net of nursing aides who usually caught patients trying to make their way back to the hall of offices. Not infrequently I heard complaints from the aides that my patients (specifically my addict patients) were too loud. Every few months I was hauled into the clinic manager's office to account for my patients' disruptions. I blushed, standing in front of the manager (her room had a faint sick smell of peppermint and dog), and told her I would sternly remind my patients of the clinic's rules.

Lucy sat stiffly in her chair. I came over to her and read the attached warnings aloud: May cause drowsiness. Alcohol intensifies effect. Use care if operating machinery. May cause dizziness. Taking more than recommended dose may cause breathing problems.

I ripped through the bag and removed the small bottle, with six tablets rattling inside. I untwisted the white safety cap, shook out two, and handed them to her. "Here's what you do. You take these two back out to the waiting area and put them under your tongue. Don't swallow them. You let your saliva pool and don't talk. It will take about ten minutes for the pills to melt and get fully liquefied. Don't be in a rush. If you don't wait for them to soak in and absorb, you won't get the full effect. You'll start feeling better within the hour. I'll have you sit in the waiting room for twenty minutes after the pills are gone. After that, we can talk briefly again in my office and then you can go."

Buprenorphine has a sweet, nasty taste that makes patients want to spit it out fast. But hurrying, not waiting for the pills to dissolve and get absorbed, leads to a mistaken underestimation of its potency.

I could have sent Lucy home with her medicine and these instructions, but I wanted to make sure she was feeling better before she left. I wanted her to connect me with improvement, instead of the torture of the last fourteen hours.

I also wanted to be certain the buprenorphine did not make her feel worse. Worsening could only happen in one instance: if she had lied and taken her final Vicodin within the last few hours before she arrived rather than at 6:00 P.M. yesterday as I instructed. If that was true, the buprenorphine would not relieve symptoms, but would precipitate them. I have seen patients experience a full withdrawal over the course of twenty minutes, ending with vomiting and muscle spasms. It is upsetting to watch, and heart-wrenching.

The idea that she could leave the premises in thirty minutes seemed to cheer her.

"That's it?" She laughed in a vexed way.

"That's it."

I handed her the pills, which she popped under her tongue. I held on to the bottle containing the remaining tablets. I walked her out to the waiting area and pointed to an empty seat.

"No talking, please," I said. "I'll come find you in a half hour or so."

She hunched in her seat in the corner and although several kids were playing hide-and-seek in the waiting area, and several parents were yelling for them to stop, I could see that Lucy wanted to keep the world away from her until she was through this.

At this time, I was the only one of my eleven colleagues who prescribed buprenorphine. The time involved with this first medication visit, segmenting the appointment over several hours—an exam, followed by the prescription mission, the explanation of how to use the pills, the waiting to see an effect, the reevaluation—disrupted the flow of a usual morning of patients. But this was not the only reason my colleagues hesitated. Addicts were complicated and distressing. They did not behave themselves. They lied. My colleagues saw their addicted patients as excessive: too many missed visits, excuses, phone calls, requests for special treatment. Doctors tire quickly of addicts and who can blame them? Other patients skip pills and don't take advice (on average, high cholesterol and high blood pressure patients take only about half of their prescribed pills over a year), but addicts are emblems of failure and doctors don't tolerate failure very well. Most of my colleagues spent as little time with addicts as possible, transferring them to other doctors like me as quickly as they could.

After I told one of my colleagues about Dan, he said, "If he came into my office and tried that shit with me, I would have kicked him out and told him not to come back. Simple. I don't get how you put up with the bunch of them." Addicts arrive with demands and agitation and a frequent inability to be engaged in civil conversation. Addicts are bullies and contaminate us with their atrocities. I know all too well how awful addicts can be; I have to find something else in them, something thankful and sympathetic.

Many patients complain that doctors are cold, impersonal, detached. But the doctors I know all have a great deal of empathy, and none of us remember ever being taught, back in medical school, to keep a distance. Over the years, I've come to understand that a doctor's detachment is actually a moral code. It is a way to make certain that we treat everyone equally. We work at a remove, with friendly restraint, mechanically, offering new patients a cool, polite reception as a matter of evenhandedness. If and when they connect with us, then we reach out more openly on their behalf.

Thirty minutes later when I led Lucy back to my office she somehow looked smaller, hollow-cheeked and fragile.

"How are you feeling?" I asked. I expected her to be upbeat and grateful. The return of painlessness signifies a return of luck for patients. After these initial buprenorphine tablets, patients often smile for the first time—even those who have been the most unpleasant, uncooperative, and belligerent.

"Good enough to leave." She shrugged very slightly, sounding disappointed. Why wouldn't she look at me? She turned her head to the window. She sat defensively, as if she were trying to get away from any interaction with me. I had the feeling I often had with addicts: if I asked too many things, it could lead to disaster. Often buprenorphine patients don't feel better for some days after the initiation of therapy.

"You have four pills left in the bottle. I'd recommend taking the first two within the next couple of hours and saving the last two for later in the day. You take them the same way you did out there. Let them sit under your tongue. Don't rush or you won't absorb the medication and get its full effect," I said for the second time. "You should feel better and better as the day goes on, but you're likely to feel different from the way you've felt for a long time, so don't be surprised. Tomorrow and the next day, you'll come back and tell me if you're having any new symptoms and we'll adjust the dose as needed. Are you still planning to go to South Carolina to see your parents?"

"Yep."

She was desperate to leave. Her silence was a form of self-removal. I knew we would talk more in the visits to follow. I understood that beyond any remaining withdrawal symptoms, which should have been abating, she was finding it difficult to deliver herself into my care.

"How are you getting home today?"

"I have a ride."

My office is built for two. I like it full, not empty. I escape the sadness of caring for one patient by caring for the next. I glanced at my schedule to see who was coming in after Lucy.

I would see her the following day to ask how the first day of buprenorphine had been, and then six days later, the next Monday, in order to fiddle with her dose, the total milligrams. Everything in medicine is offered in clear units—in milligrams and deciliters—exact, categorized, numeric, which gives me the sensation of clear thinking. I again instructed Lucy to spread the four remaining pills across the day. Although buprenorphine lasts for more than twenty-four hours in the body, and thus, pharmacologically, needs to be taken only once a day (some individuals only need to use it every other day), Vicodin addicts are used to taking thirty pills a day, every four to six hours. Putting a pill into their mouths throughout the day has become routine, and they often feel better using buprenorphine twice or even three times a day, breaking pills in half so that they feel they have more available later if they need it. It is a matter of control. I had given Lucy lower-strength tablets so that, cumulatively, we could determine what dose made her comfortable. But even after we settled on a standing dose, a week or two from now, I knew Lucy might well split the prescription into eight- or twelve-hour intervals as a means of psychological insurance, and this was fine by me, as long as she told me what she was doing. In a few weeks (if she continued to see me), she would feel physically well on an established dose of buprenorphine, and we would see each other less frequently over the next months.

Sobriety is fragile, elusive. I wanted Lucy to try to live as if she didn't have a drug problem. As if she could be a person not marked by drugs. As if she didn't *have* to be thinking about Vicodin all day, but instead could wonder if Vicodin was even worth thinking about. As if there were things desirable in life outside Vicodin. To give up Vicodin was to shed the illusion that life was fine and to take on what might be another illusion: that life could be better.

Not every addict has the same goals when they come to see me. Some want to stop opiates for good, unsure whether they would need buprenorphine indefinitely or would be able to stop treatment after a short time. Some want to take a break from chasing down a source of OxyContin, Percocet, or heroin, but only expect to use buprenorphine as a temporary reprieve. Others want to reduce their use of illegal opiates, but continue at a lower level, supplemented by the buprenorphine I gave them. Of course, no addict admits to these latter options. They all tell me they want to be free of the drug permanently. Most addicts can't distinguish their real wishes from their unfulfilled ones, but then, who can?

My primary goal for this first week with Lucy had been merely to make our visits as pleasant as possible, so she felt comfortable and glad to take refuge. I wanted to spoil her with hearty welcomes and congratulations on another Vicodin-free day, so we could get on to the difficult subject of what was actually important to her. My goal was to reawaken her interest in life.

CHAPTER 4

Monday, April 28

During my second-year courses when I was in medical school in the 1980s, the drugs of addiction were described as the medications that connected us to the doctors of antiquity. *Papaver somniferum,* the sleep-inducing poppy with the pod of opium, was familiar to Arab, Greek, and Roman physicians who had always been interested in psychoactive drugs. Systematically cultivated for eighty-five hundred years in Mesopotamia, this "plant of joy" was used over the centuries as an aphrodisiac, as a sedative for troublesome children, as a healer of liver complaints, scorpion bites, and elephantiasis and also during religious ceremonies. It even played a role in overtaking thrones. Nero poisoned Britannicus with opiates.

Our sideburned professor of pharmacology offered us a short history of laudanum—opium tincture in alcohol—dosed by the dropperful (De Quincey, author of *Confessions of an English Opium Eater,* used eight thousand drops a day). Laudanum was a cure-all from the Enlightenment onward, where ever-hopeful, but increasingly circumspect, physicians found it didn't do much good for fevers or sexual potency, measles, or seizures; but it did allay pain, improve coughs, and check diarrhea, all of which opiates were still used for. Our professor showed us pictures of cakes of dark brown opium, which had been baked that very year in Afghanistan to the consistency of clay. It was being abundantly trafficked and was part of an estimated 10 percent of the total produced annually that was hotly pursued by police in the West, who did not welcome it as the drug of joy. His larger point was that culturally we have always been preoccupied with drugs. Caffeine was outlawed in the seventeenth century as a cause of physical and emotional deterioration. Germans felt that tobacco use should be punishable by death after its first appearance, and in nineteenth-century Russia, castration was fitting for users. Coffee drinkers and smokers were seen as willful, uncontrollable, threatening.

Although we learned some history and policy in pharmacology class, we also were trained to calculate equivalent doses of opiate derivatives—how milligrams of morphine could be translated in milligrams of Dilaudid or Demerol. We were taught the names of the receptors in the brain where these chemicals connected (all narcotics attached to mu receptors, which were densely concentrated in the parts of the brain that modulated pleasure), and how long each opiate lasted in the body before it was metabolized. We briefly discussed what happened when a patient overdosed or experienced drug withdrawal, and all told, this instruction took a mere two hours during two years of classroom training.

I wish my medical school coursework had better prepared me to care for a patient dependent on narcotics, but it didn't. In all the patient case studies I heard discussed during my training—a women with acute kidney failure after a radiological procedure, an old man with a heart murmur and bounding pulses, a young women with acutely swollen joints, a rash, and a fever—I was never presented with a "Dan" who came in with pain that I could neither confirm nor diagnose. A man who, cloaked in bitterness and guile, asked me for a specific addictive pill. We never discussed how patients might end their drug use behaviors or how, as physicians, we might help. That was the work of drug counselors, who worked in specialized treatment programs quite apart from the medical system; social workers; mutual help groups like Narcotics Anonymous; or finally, because the outcome was nearly hopeless, ministers. As a student, I had the typical layperson's view of drug addiction: it wasn't something you slipped in and out of; once you became an addict, you were always an addict. It was permanent.

There was a weeklong unit that concerned the many clinical effects of alcohol. All of us knew something about liquor: its smell, the lovely sound of a wineglass being filled, the rush and foam of a plastic dorm-room cup held under a keg tap. Alcohol was ubiquitous, bought by our parents and given as presents. It was never *not there*—on the counter next to the coffeemaker, in the refrigerator, at parties. We knew so many people who drank alcohol, and such a small proportion were identifiably alcoholic, we thought these few must have had extenuating circumstances that explained their dependence. Even after a week of lectures, hardly any of us—except those who had an alcoholic relative—had a sense of how one "became" alcohol dependent, that it could be subtle and insidious and involved denial long after the fact.

The simple advice to a heavy-drinking patient was *drink less*; could a doctor really say the same to a heroin user, *use less*, knowing that being caught with *any* could put you in prison, that even a single injection could be life-threatening?

I was first exposed to the clinical consequences of opiate addiction as a third-year medical student on the wards of Harlem Hospital. This was during the height of the HIV era, and heroin injectors were coming in with odd infections and dying in a matter of days. Those who didn't have AIDS were admitted with simpler and curable maladies like subcutaneous abscesses and skin infections. Despite their grossly swollen hands or legs, they felt luckier than their friends and drug partners who were a few beds away waiting to die "from the virus." And they weren't shy to talk, either. "I'll talk to you and I won't even ask you to pay me," one patient said early in my rotation. I was an easy mark, a young white male in a short white coat.

A medical student's challenge is to be helpful when feeling helpless. All medical students are aware of their shortcomings, and I was aware of my inability to recognize certain physical findings (the distention of neck veins signaling heart failure), my amateurish way of performing an examination, and my insufficient grasp of physiology. I was also aware that the older patients on the ward often died, whereas the addicts, nearly all of whom were under thirty, were more likely to get out alive. I found it easier to talk to them than to manage the deaths of the patients who were my grandparents' age. At the same time, I was being exposed to an America I'd never been a part of, and I had the sense of learning about another world just by sitting with addicts.

I was incapable of impressing teachers with my knowledge, but compensated by being kind to my patients. I doted on the heroin users by bringing them graham crackers and orange juice.

I got their TVs switched on and covered them with extra blankets when they were rolled to tests. I could not think of a single reason not to give them what they asked for. I didn't know enough to be wary. I knew their behavior could be rough, but I never felt it. Given their lives on the street, it was amazing how few addicts were violently confrontational. Nurses and respiratory technicians and physical therapists would complain that my addict-patients would scream and spit and throw pills when they felt insulted or cheated or mistreated. But I was never the subject of their ire.

The addicts were young and loud and called me "rookie." We were friendly, but I never forgot they were criminals, with Rikers and Sing Sing behind and in front of them. I was new to it all, and not a longtime, third-shift nurse who, after twenty years, couldn't stand much of anything that caused extra work. I could tell it was hard for a lot of the staff to be polite to the addicts.

On the men's wards, I was a few years younger than they were, but I was interested in music, and this brought us oddly close. I had time, I was available, and what fully formed doctor wanted to talk with them? In four-bed rooms the addicts colluded and joked and invited me to play cards and dominoes. They didn't mind the laziness of hospital life, the lounging around in green foam slippers. But they were existentially unhappy—I knew because of the dull distress I felt when I got home, the anguish when I recalled listening to the one addict who dragged his IV pole every afternoon to the phone booth to call his mother, asking about his brother hospitalized in Brooklyn also for a drug-related infection. I had the sense the addicts had nothing to hurry back to outside, no immediate tasks to get done.

Conversation was a form of play, of relaxation that was meant to make a young doctor-in-training smile. The sniffers showed me how to slice a straw, and the injectors introduced me to their monstrous rituals: the licking of the needle tip, the anticipatory tapping of the vein, the blood clouding the clear heroin solution in the syringe when they pulled back on the plunger to check if a vein had been entered. They taught me about veins that they used when the obvious ones on the hands, wrists, and forearms were sclerosed—next to the pulse at the groin, under the tongue, inside the eyelid, along the top of an erection. They shared the names of their bagged and bundled (ten bags to a bundle, ten dollars a bag) products—Poison and Homicide and No Way Out and Mercy— the wordplay of clever branding.

They spoke as though it was all a code to understanding plea- sure. They'd say, "You try it the first time and all you think is when you can do it again." Getting high offered more than a moment of exultation; it stretched time and was a way of slowing things down and bringing them into focus. Heroin was a way to shape the day, set a schedule. Its chemistry was an alarm clock set at six- to eight-hour intervals. You knew what you needed and when, predictably, without surprises. It gave you what you were expecting; what was promised was delivered. Heroin was an occupation and a motivation. It gave structure to structure-less lives.

I said hardly anything, heard a lot, and tended to believe most of it. Around the addicts, I felt oversized, clumsy, constrained, naive. From their invitations, they must have had some sense I was attracted to their worst sides—the dishonest, devious, angry, and disgraced sides, the ones willing to be at the mercy of desire.

They were "hooked" on heroin. The sharp need for the next dose was buried in their flesh. Stuck, caught, damaged, hooked. Some asked to be freed, but not one asked for exculpation or forgiveness. No addict thought heroin was heroic, but they didn't think it was evil, either. They knew it was dangerous. This was the underside, the wreckage of the booming American 1980s. America was shining and these were the shamed, the ones who kept out of sight. AIDS was rampant among injectors in New York; their friends were dying in ways far uglier than an overdose or choking on vomit.

They were sometimes melancholy, but they were also lively and energetic compared with the old women with heart disease and old men with emphysema. Years later, I remembered how immensely satisfying the work with addicts was, their brain-teasing diagnoses, how much pleasure I got when I figured out that they could find their own veins better than I could. Why *not* let them draw their own blood in the morning? I secretly handed out needles and purple-topped tubes and tourniquets at 8:00 A.M. and came back a half hour later to pick them up, handing the blood samples over to my superiors as if I were an expert phlebotomist. If my patients led unconventional lives, why couldn't I?

If I had worked these early medical school ward months in the suburbs rather than in Harlem, my clinical interest might have taken a different direction. At Harlem Hospital, I met a class of people I'd never met before, who lived on the edge of my awareness: parking lot attendants, wig store workers, toll collectors, security guards, cashiers, home health aides, bookies. The urban poor, humble, unsure of their worth. The life of the addict seemed so closely bound up with the life of the city. And when I walked out the front door of the hospital onto the street, I loved watching the unsteady crowd in front of the liquor store, the broken glass on the sidewalks, the sneakers strung over the telephone wires, the aesthetic of disaster. I trained my eye to be receptive to swollen hands and track-marked arms, furious itching and runny noses, and would watch for this on people in the subway. This exposure to addiction foreshadowed my later interests. My buprenorphine patients are still house painters and carpet layers, clam diggers and guitarists without gigs, short-order cooks and funeral directors, as well as an occasional lawyer or mortgage broker. Some use heroin, some use pills.

I graduated from medical school as an optimist. I believed in second chances (even for addicts who really hadn't had a first chance). An addict's fall from grace might be temporary, I thought. Much of my current desire to prescribe buprenorphine can probably be traced back to falling under the spell of my first patients at Harlem Hospital, who, it went without saying, had few treatment options. I still remember the addict who, after lying for twelve hours in the corner of the emergency room withdrawing from heroin, asked me, "What kind of doctor are you?" And I remember finally understanding that he was really asking, "What kind of person are you?"

Lucy was neither friendly nor unfriendly when she came into my office that Monday—a week after I'd first given her buprenorphine—but she was alert, in the way addicts always are, no matter how sleepy or troubled she appeared. She was wearing drab clothes, thrift shop vintage, a little faded, a little dirty, inauspicious; she was an early morning mess, and seemed to be clutching her white lidless coffee cup. Her eyes danced, but her long legs moved slowly. She had made it through a week.

"It's been a bad few days," she said, almost in a whisper. She shuffled to her chair, and sat with her legs hung over one metal arm of the chair, shaping her into an N. Her facial muscles tightened.

"In what way?" I asked. I knew it was impossible for her to reconstruct how her mind had been working through her drug problem.

"I've just been feeling bad. But I'm leaving for South Carolina soon," she added, trying to be cheerful. She had a single worry wrinkle across her forehead.

She leaned over to put her coffee cup on the floor and, still seated, twisted herself out of her long blue peacoat. She looked for somewhere to put it and laid it on the floor beside her chair, then reached again for her coffee, her hand shaking a bit. She looked caught, confused, ashamed. As usual, she gave me her profile; she was looking elsewhere.

"The second day I saw you, I called Brian from downstairs as soon as I left. I told him, 'I'm sick.'"

I'd seen her the morning after the initial dosing visit. The worst of withdrawal was already in the past, I'd assumed. She looked well when she walked out of my office on the day of the first dose. "The buprenorphine I gave you made you sick?" I was surprised.

Blocking withdrawal symptoms, and with virtually no side effects of its own, buprenorphine rarely makes patients sick during the first days. At the second visit, I had given her buprenorphine for six additional days, enough to get her through the weekend until today.

"It sure did. I'd used Vicodin late during the night I first saw you. You'd given me two extra pills for Tuesday and I used them a few hours after I left you that day, but they put me into horrible withdrawal."

I'd warned her not to go back and forth between Vicodin and buprenorphine, but she'd done exactly what I'd told her not to do. I like to think of myself as open to hearing whatever a patient told me, but maybe I hadn't been when she returned on day two of buprenorphine. She had used Vicodin without thinking, without feeling she had a choice because it was what she'd been doing every day for years; she must have felt there was no escape except to continue, even when I'd handed her an escape in the form of buprenorphine. Now I was discouraged by the way she sat sideways in her chair, her back curled. I was discouraged by her bad posture, her adolescent slump. I was discouraged that she had disregarded my advice. She was causing *herself* trouble while inescapable misery came to other patients for no reason at all (my last patient had been a forty-three-year-old man with pancreatic cancer). I didn't see an approved mechanism to ensure success with Lucy or Julia or Tom. Did their lives depend on what happened in my office? Maybe. The profession of medicine thrives on the perpetual expectation of change for the better (that is the point of round after horrendous round of cancer chemotherapy), and over the years I had assumed this as my natural attitude, even with addicts.

Whenever we made unwanted eye contact, Lucy raised her eyebrows and rolled her lips inward.

"Brian was not happy that I was sick. He was out trying to make some money. He found this abandoned fertilizer factory that was about to be torn down out in the country and he's been ripping metal from the building, stripping it. We park outside and load up the car. I help him take the easy stuff first, tubing, copper wire, stainless steel. He sells it as scrap metal. We can hardly breathe inside there's so much formaldehyde. Have you ever seen formaldehyde? It looks like ice flowing out of those tanks. The whole place is bright blue from the fertilizer. When I called Brian and told him I was sick, he was pissed that I was bothering him. 'How sick?' he asked me. 'Really sick. I can't drive. I've got to get out of here,' I told him. He picked me up with the car full of formaldehyde-coated metal. The car seats were blue from the dust.

"I don't know if it was the smell in the car or because of the buprenorphine, but I was throwing up out the window the whole ride home. Brian left me in the apartment and sold the stuff he'd collected that day for three hundred bucks, but it felt like a long time before he came home with more Vicodin for me."

He probably spent the $300 on himself, I thought. I am always surprised when I hear that an addict runs out of drugs. Why do they? They know the routine. Can they not afford more than a day or two? Do they avoid having too many pills lying around because their friends might steal them? Do they believe they might quit in the next few days? Do they let themselves run out as a form of self-punishment?

"And the next day?" I asked her. "Did you go back on the buprenorphine?"

One of my colleagues believes that most patients say what they need to say for him to make a full diagnosis in the first few sentences of the visit. And if he interrupts with questions early on, he can winnow his initial list of possible diagnoses efficiently and accurately, and won't miss much except for irrelevant refinements and emotional wanderings (the parts of a visit I often find most absorbing). Caring for addicts, I have found that the exact opposite technique holds the only hope of figuring out what is going on. The gist of the problem does not come out in the first words, or early on, or even until a second or third or fourth visit, as seemed the case with Lucy. Addicts hide things—they keep secrets for years, decades. Just because they are expected to divulge their symptoms and actions doesn't mean they will.

"I came here for my pills the second day, but I was still using Vicodin. I used what Brian bought me on that day, then $100 worth to stop me from throwing up on Wednesday, but it didn't help, so I bought $200 worth on Thursday, and I still didn't feel good. I'd sleep for a couple of hours, but mostly I was up watching TV. That made me feel a little better."

In one week Lucy had established the pattern I see too often with my patients. At each visit, I give exactly enough buprenorphine to get them back to the next visit with no pills remaining. But on some days patients use more than prescribed, some days less. If a patient approaches the next visit with a few pills left, she'll hide them, save them, in case some day I cut her off, or she has to go out of town unexpectedly. If a patient comes up short, he is out of luck unless he borrows from a friend or buys buprenorphine on the street. Most such patients go back to the drug they are trying to quit.

I remembered looking and listening on Tuesday for clues, nuances in Lucy's speech, that might have tipped me to her continued Vicodin use. I'd directly asked if she was still using, but she had an easy duplicity. Truth was a compromise, a matter of degree. She'd looked at me in surprise, as if I should have known better, before replying, "Of course not." She hid things well in her blue eyes. *Never again.* Addicts say it all the time. They smile and say it, voices filled with emotion.

Maybe this was how Lucy thought the world conducted itself. Half-secret, half-open, her two lives. I have never accepted any of my patients, addicts or nonaddicts, as reliable narrators. I ask them to retell the sequence of symptoms (did the cough start before the chest discomfort or vice versa?) and to attribute causality (did you wake at night because you were short of breath or did you awaken and then notice you couldn't breathe?). With each version of events they offer—and it is never the same twice—I make no gesture that signifies assent. I do not want them to believe that there is a "right" answer. Because a medical office offers an atmosphere and a relationship different from any other, I have heard my colleagues question whether a doctor's office could ever really be the "real world" to patients. But I have no doubt about this: I represent reality *fully* apprehended, which explains why patients sometimes choose not to mention the odd mole they'd noticed between their fourth and fifth toes, or the chest discomfort they had when they raked leaves, until well into our time together; they are scared. They don't want bad news. They aren't trying to deceive, but their stories contain unconscious biases, hopeful reframings, counterphobic oversights.

There was no denying that Lucy had deliberately not told me about her continued Vicodin use. It wasn't careless. Did she enjoy this drama? Did she think of us as antagonists, in opposition? I didn't believe so. She had tried to figure out what I wanted to hear, and supplied it, while she went about her personal pharmacological experiment (*what if I use buprenorphine then Vicodin? what if I use Vicodin then buprenorphine?*). Many opiate users test the strength and activity of buprenorphine, wanting to understand how it works *in them*, just as they have been interested in every pill they've ever swallowed. Some consider such pill-mixing perverse. But I expect most addicts to mix as they please. I understood how Lucy could continue to use Vicodin and yet return to see me wanting to continue in the program.

Her on-again, off-again withdrawal symptoms from taking buprenorphine and Vicodin together seemed to have caused worse problems. I was glad it had taken her only a week to trust me with the news. I presumed she was fighting to get better, she wanted to get better, but perhaps she'd lost her forward progress; she wasn't proud. Sometimes patients lie—my appetite was much better this week, I've been sleeping very well—because they want to fool themselves; they feel another bad day coming. Medical therapy is founded on forward motion, steady improvement, and we are all loathe to acknowledge its failure. Having seen too many addicts over the years, maybe I accept their slipperiness and inadequacies too peacefully. Maybe Lucy needed to deal with Brian in a certain way and she had a habit of omission that carried over into my office. Maybe I was simply born believing that whenever a patient tells a story about herself, to some degree she is making it up.

Lying has a tremendous power to drive people away, doctors in particular. To protect our patients from being labeled liars, to give them dignity again, to reimagine our role, we call a patient's lying "denial." Denial, as one of addiction's chief symptoms, has lying as its legacy. Many of the addicts in my office are inept, unlucky, or unsuccessful in their lives, and so they fabricate preposterous tales about their accomplishments, good fortune, achievements. They are definite about everything, but can document nothing. They lie about new clothes and new cars and big jobs. They pull things from their pockets to show me: cash, keys, jewels, lottery tickets. They talk fast, their mouths dry. Addicts are always about to "get something" from somebody, a ride, a check, a new apartment. They pretend to have hurt feelings if I doubt them, ask them to explain more. Not everyone can tell a decent lie.

With some of my elderly patients, I am willing to wink or smile or eye-roll in sympathy with their make-believe stories. But I keep a serious face on for addicts. My expression is meant to be respectful, but skeptical. It is meant to convey that this is a serious business we are discussing—the risk of incarceration, family destruction, overdose and suicide. A straight face lets me keep on message, and the message is: many bad things have already happened to you, and worse is possible, even if you don't admit this to me or yourself.

With Dan, the truth wasn't of much use. Lies were an integral part of his language—what he'd done, where he'd been. If he'd accepted my ten-pill plan, he probably would have been back fifteen minutes later telling me, "You forgot to give me the prescription," or two hours later with, "That wasn't me you gave a prescription to, it must have been some other patient." He exaggerated, he concocted. His reports didn't hang together. They were unverifiable. In a single visit with Dan I'd seen that some of his lies came solemnly, others with a nervous laugh. Caught, he would have been unrepentant.

If Lucy hadn't already told me, I would have eventually found out that she had continued to use Vicodin through a urine test. But now I didn't need to bother with a urine collection.

When addicts are motivated and feeling well, they walk in saying, "I'm ready to give a urine today." They can't wait to start showing me proof of their clean living. They are proud of themselves for a week of drug-free existence. Sometimes I could just look at them and say, "I don't need a sample today, my guess is you're doing just fine." But sometimes they insist, as if they want to take a printout of the lab results home to frame. Often they don't realize that marijuana shows up a month later in a toxicology and that their report card might not be so perfect. The sleeping pill borrowed the night before from a brother-in-law, which they didn't even think of as an addictive substance, shows up, too. But for patients taking buprenorphine, the marijuana and Xanax aren't pertinent; only the "Opiates Negative" line matters to them.

Was Lucy really *"tired"* of Vicodin and ready to quit? Or was she planning to continue it right through her trip to South Carolina with buprenorphine serving as backup in case she ran out of Vics when she was there? Was she playing me? Narcotics are a nearly invincible, overwhelming force, and addiction is a form of love: in the way it unsettles, in the way it causes pain, in the way it disturbs the ordinary emotional tenor of life. It takes a leap of faith to quit; a change of heart feels hopeless.

"For some reason I still believe that I could have a meaningful life."

That's what she said at her first visit. I was glad Lucy had told me about her Vicodin use, even if it was a week late.

There was something sweet and open and self-mocking about her confession. Her expression appeared to say, *Look at all this trouble I've caused myself. We both know I'm a little crazy, but please believe me when I tell you I mean to quit.* She was oddly naive; she hadn't calculated the possible implications of her lies. She didn't seem to understand that using Vicodin in addition to buprenorphine jeopardized her continuation in the program, that I didn't *have* to give her any more buprenorphine. I could have decided that the buprenorphine had failed for Lucy, and I should rethink whether this was the best treatment for her.

It was not obstinacy that kept her using; I was more positive-minded than that. I wasn't ready to dismiss her. I don't mind that my work with some patients involves steadfastness and persistence, a three-steps backward, one-forward approach. Maybe I'd picked this up from the addicts I worked with in Harlem, the ones who were rehospitalized three or four times in the few months I was there. I didn't mind keeping vigil as Lucy tried to improve. I liked that she needed me. But she needed to stay away from certain things and certain people, and Brian, I thought, was a problem for her. When I thought of Lucy and Brian, I thought of disorder.

"So after three days of taking Vicodin to stop you from throwing up, and having realized that mixing it with the pills I gave you was *causing* you to throw up, what did you do?" I asked again. I tried not to sound harsh.

She sipped her coffee. She hid behind it. She gulped. Then she put it down again under her chair. I didn't drink coffee, but I liked the smell taking over the room.

"I realized I had to stop one or the other. I realized I was making it worse by mixing the buprenorphine and the Vicodin. I was so sick I was hoping against hope that the next pill, whichever it was, would make me feel better."

Every day an addict uses, she feels like she's cheating at something. Even if she believes she will never get caught or in trouble, she knows she's cheating. This cheating had literally made Lucy sick. She had experimented with combining pills since she was a teenager, so I wasn't surprised by her admission. I'd given her the schedule and rules of the program on day one: *Don't lose your medications if you expect me to give you more. Don't skip appointments.* The conditions of treatment were clear (but didn't include the commandment, Thou shalt never use opiates again), and it would have been indelicate to bring them up again. I'd learned that when I was calm, my patients were, too.

"Brian was stealing my Vicodin, and taking some of my buprenorphine as well. 'Why shouldn't I try them?' he said to me, 'You're sick already.'

"He doesn't care about me. I was sick and he was sending me out for cookies and grape soda and Big Macs. He'd tell me, 'I left some Vics sitting in the dish on the counter for you.' But they weren't there when I got home. 'We must have been robbed,' he said. He was pissed I wasn't going to work so he would have money for his lottery numbers. He's incapable of caring about me. I called my mother in South Carolina and asked her to buy me that plane ticket."

Was her mother ready to take care of her sick daughter, ready to bring the cool washcloth and lay it across her forehead? I wasn't sure.

I had been wondering since Lucy's first visit what her parents knew about her life these days. She had originally said that if her mother knew the details she "would drop dead on the spot." She had proudly described them as two people with advanced academic degrees. I remembered thinking that the mention of the graduate school degrees, the display of her parents' intellectual credentials was a shorthand for the expectations they had had for her.

Her parents didn't know her life now, but what about when she was living with them? She had started using drugs as a young teenager, and I could imagine her parents going through the house as I would have, searching for what she'd hidden, yanking open drawers, looking under the mattress, sweating, afraid of what they'd find. But more than once Lucy had described her mother's powers of denial as being incredibly impressive. I wondered if that was true, or if her mother simply never mentioned those moments of terror when she uncovered pill bottles, cans, glassine envelopes, paper bags.

"My mother was thrilled that I wanted to visit them in South Carolina, if I haven't made that clear. She was waiting for me to call back before she bought the ticket. I haven't even been there. I know, from what I told you before, that it must seem like my family neglected me, but the opposite is true."

She sat up in her chair, slid down again.

"And how many more days can I stay in and watch Burt Reynolds movies? I love them, all of them, the police ones, the romances. They're not good movies, but it's not as if they *tried* to be good and failed. I don't know why I like them so much. I must identify them as seventies movies or something. Last night, I did my antisocial thing, and watched *The Cannonball Run*."

"And Brian?"

"He still doesn't believe I'm going to South Carolina. I'm not sure I believe it after my call this morning. I was on the phone with my mother, and my father was screaming at her in the background the entire time. He's fifty-five years old, he wants a motorboat, and he claims she's interfering. My father invents reasons to scream at her. It's been a long time since I've seen him, but this was pretty typical.

"The last time I was there, the motorboat thing had him storming in and out of house. For three years it's been going on. He puts down a deposit and withdraws it. He puts down another and withdraws it again. Meanwhile, he tells her not to buy a new car, even though hers breaks down every other week. She can drive his when he gets his boat, he says. If your precious daughter needs a ride anywhere, rent a car, I heard him scream. When he got on the phone the last time and I tried to make conversation, asking him about the motorboat quest, he spit, 'None of that is happening. Not now.'

"One minute she makes excuses for his screaming—'he needs to see someone for mental health help'—the next minute he's the dream husband. Growing up, one minute I heard, 'Don't end up with someone like your father.' The next day it was like she never said it. I don't know what possessed her to stay with him all these years."

"So there will be plenty of stress in the house when you get there."

"I've spent my whole life anxious. I'm used to it."

"But you've never taken any medication for anxiety, is that right?"

"Taking a medicine that isn't Vicodin has never been a high priority for me," she said with a flash of insight that again made me hopeful. "My mother said she was going to invite my sister down from Chicago."

"Is that good news or bad news?"

"She probably won't come. She's too busy with her job and her serious boyfriend. She and I were never close, not even as kids.

We didn't fight, but we weren't close. I guess we had different interests: Robin was normal. She was into sports, and she never did as well as I did in school before I stopped going. She was *too* well adjusted. She was happy everywhere she went. She never caused my parents problems. She didn't relate to me, and to be fair, I didn't relate to her. I never had much to do with her. By the time I was fifteen, I had a boyfriend in college anyway. He was one of the nicer guys I ever went out with. My taste has gotten progressively worse.

"When my mother had lymphoma, after she had chemo, her liver failed. My sixteen-year-old sister refused to visit the hospital. I stayed with my mother in the hospital, but I never cried and I felt guilty that I wasn't taking her impending death harder."

Outside, I could see a bent-over man who was raking. The grass of his small front yard was brown. He'd converted the two strips along the curb to wood chips so he wouldn't have to reseed in the spring.

"My mother was on a ventilator for a month, a good part of that in a coma. I was living at home that summer with my father, who was hell. All he did was yell and scream. But in this one case my father's stubbornness paid off. They kept asking him to take her off the ventilator and he refused. Just after she got out of the hospital, I went back to school and took some of her Vicodin with me.

"Sometimes I wish they'd disown me," Lucy went on. "But they won't. They do the opposite, torture me with their demands and high hopes. I'm jealous of people from lower-class families who have no expectations. Brian's family is a mess. His sister married a homeless man, for God's sake."

She forced herself to smile and shake her head.

"With me leaving for South Carolina, Brian started talking this morning about cleaning up. Two addicts in the same apartment trying to quit at the same time. Now *there's* an impossibility."

I presumed everyone in her world, Brian's world, copped drugs, shared drugs, perhaps sold them. Every acquaintance Lucy had probably used, and although it was acceptable not to use for a while, opiates influenced every relationship, romance, roommate situation. Before Brian there had been other men who used opiates, who sat around watching TV, working occasionally, while she held this or that job for three or four months to pay for her share of the drugs.

Brian had recently talked about methadone treatment, and she could have chosen that instead of buprenorphine. Methadone is another long-acting, synthetic drug that works on the same brain receptors as buprenorphine. Available since the 1960s, federal regulations dictated that methadone could only be prescribed for opiate dependence by doctors working at licensed centers; by law, I had never written a methadone prescription to treat addiction. The year before, Brian had been enrolled in one of six centers in the city. Guided by a strict set of rules and therefore dependent on bureaucratic structure, methadone programs required seven-day-a-week medication visits during the initial months of treatment. Each morning, patients formed winding lines and one by one approached a glass booth where they ingested the daily liquid dose, orange-colored, pumped from an industrial-sized dispenser, and served in a thimble-sized paper cup.

Every methadone program in our city is still housed in a run-down neighborhood, in a nondescript building with caged windows and steel doors marked with no logo. The sidewalk outside is littered with cigarette butts and gum and fast-food wrappers. Addicts arrive with certain low expectations and they are met. "Counseling" is mandated at all programs. Nationally, most counselors are former addicts with little training; although some are talented, fewer than half are licensed. (Licenses do not require a bachelor's degree and can be received in under six months.) It is a lower level of accreditation than anywhere else in health care, acceptable, some might say, only because the patients are addicts, and they don't have a lobby in Washington. Many think they don't deserve any treatment at all. Imagine if depression counseling in America was offered only by people recently depressed, none of whom had been to graduate school to learn the well-studied dos and don'ts of skillful psychological treatment and specific protocols that might work best.

Methadone works for those who stick with it. It has been available to treat opiate dependence for forty years before buprenorphine, and the research on methadone treatment has repeatedly demonstrated its efficacy in decreasing drug use—preventing deaths, HIV infection, incarceration for selling or using drugs—and increasing the return of addicts to work and family and functional life during the time they remain on methadone. In addition, some methadone programs medicate you on the day you arrive for treatment, an advantage over the waiting period of my buprenorphine protocol.

At the time I was seeing Lucy, the cost of methadone treatment was right, even if it was not covered by insurance—and in many places it wasn't. Standard doses of methadone wholesaled at under fifty cents a day, lower than many prescribed medications in America. Because most programs were franchises (part of national for-profit chains that tracked client census), had minimal overhead, and paid counselors poorly, prices were kept low so that addicts could pay cash, often not more than $75 a week for the counseling, urine testing, and medication.

Nonetheless, it was obvious why Lucy might favor the more

expensive buprenorphine (ten bucks a day for medication alone, plus medical visits, plus toxicologies). Even if my waiting area was an exhausting, crowded, multilingual human whirlpool, she got to sit with other patients who *weren't* addicts. It was a relief to get into my office for a regularly scheduled doctor's appointment, a medical visit that could be understood by friends, employers, parents. She could have been coming to see me for any medical problem; that was all people had to know.

I'd recently referred Marco to a methadone program after I'd prescribed buprenorphine for six months. Marco had come in addicted to OxyContin. He was about to lose his job as a cook and I remembered the first day he walked in wearing a knee-to-neck white chef's tunic, its square collar as high and tight as a straitjacket. He was having no trouble finding Oxys among the kitchen staff and was spending two hundred bucks for two hundred milligrams a day, which he needed to get through lunch and dinner in the kitchen without having withdrawal symptoms. He understood that my program's goal is abstinence and he swore he could do it. For a month, he was OxyContin free on buprenorphine. But then he started delivering opiate-positive urines, as well as a series of excuses about life stresses and setbacks. I was lenient; he had a wife and a new baby he didn't want to disappoint. He was a handsome man of thirty-three, cocky, high-strung and enthusiastic, and he was mad about cooking. His tunic was always a splattered mess, and he wore it to every appointment, either coming from work or going there, which was an eighty-hour-a-week labor of love.

Three months into his treatment, after another unpromising urine toxicology, I dragged out the stack of results and showed him that buprenorphine hadn't allowed him to quit OxyContin. "But I'm only using on Sunday nights," he told me in his gravelly, low-sizzle voice, "at the end of my workweek. I'm celebrating. No harm done. It's better than it was when I started here."

He felt he was succeeding, and it was true that according to a weekly count of drug use days, Marco was better. By his own admission, it was clear that his goal was to manage his narcotic use, not to get it out of his life. He was hedging his bets; he wanted to have buprenorphine around, but also use Oxys from time to time.

There comes a point with many patients on buprenorphine where the primary and most easily gauged measure of treatment success, abstinence, has not been reached, and doctor and patient have to decide how to proceed. To enter my program is to make a commitment to quitting opiates, or at least a good-faith attempt. I wasn't sure that I believed Marco was using only on Sundays. I had no way to confirm this, and when he refused to bring in his wife to give another view, I became extremely doubtful. I was concerned that if he was using once a week, he would soon be using twice or three times, the inevitable escalation because OxyContin (ground up and sniffed) always felt better than buprenorphine. I warned him that he needed at least two weeks in a row of opiate-free toxicologies to continue to see me for buprenorphine.

The next visit, he again gave an opiate-positive urine. He pretended to feel bad, but I could tell he couldn't believe I was bringing up his Sunday use as a problem again. One measly day a week. He felt obliged to say he was planning to quit. I also didn't appreciate his belief that I would go on accepting his excuses forever. I had reached the point with Marco where there was no more thinking that things would be better. He knew I was unhappy.

At his last visit, I was grave, with arms folded when he came in. He looked frustrated; his brow furrowed. He wasn't like Dan who just disappeared. But Dan had seen me only once; Marco and I had sat together for nearly six months, talking about the Food Channel and the Red Sox and the price jump of postage stamps, and the war in Iraq. But it had all been filler, a way for him to avoid paying attention to his symptoms, actions, and motivations. Our previous conversations had been superficial, and that was okay because what mattered those first months were the negative toxicologies Marco managed to achieve; long-term abstinence from OxyContin, followed by a tapering off of buprenorphine, seemed within reach. Now I knew he was still in love with his opiate. He probably had a supply of buprenorphine at home from the days he'd skipped it to get high, unless he had been trading it to other kitchen staff for the OxyContin.

When I told Marco about the methadone programs in town, and how going to one of them might be the way to really be done with OxyContin because of the structured, daily oversight, he nodded, stepped back, extended his hand, and shook mine. He laugh-huffed once, not with me, but at me, another unfortunate doctor who didn't "get" it. I knew what he thought of me. But this wasn't about me.

How do old values give way to new ones? Sometimes with a push from a doctor, sometimes with a push from a spouse, and sometimes it takes a trip to jail to shake people up. I had warned Marco about his continued OxyContin use, but the rules governing my care of him were not exactly the same ones I applied to Monica, whom I continued to care for despite weekly opiate use. Of course she didn't see me for buprenorphine treatment. Neither Marco nor Monica wanted to be abstinent, but Marco wanted it both ways: to keep using OxyContin and to keep using me as his source of buprenorphine. Medical care is not catechism. It is not a memorized algorithm. It is amassed data, plus experience, leading to speculation and judgment and inconsistent practice (that can probably be defended in retrospect, but maybe not) over a series of patients.

So let me try this again: When was the last time you used Vicodin?" I asked Lucy.

"Three days ago," she said. "I'm telling you, this last week was the sickest I've ever been since I started taking drugs. I've been using only buprenorphine for three straight days now. I'm not going to use any more Vicodin because I'm not going to go through that again."

At some point, I had to accept what she said, or my treatment would never be helpful. I wanted to say to her, "Just stay Vicodin-free for a few weeks and all will be well," but it wasn't true. She had years of struggle ahead.

Patients are inconsistent and therefore changeable. The changes they make are not always conscious or done willingly. Sometimes change comes in bursts, quickly, sharply. Sometimes it proceeds very slowly. The question with Lucy remained, *What could I do to help?* I would have to work to engage her—accepting a few untruths and some opiate-positive urines during these early visits. Patients often wear me out with their theories and justifications, but I need to keep a desperate eagerness to understand what they tell, feel, and do. The trick for every doctor is not to lose interest and to find some value even in the lies. Through my eagerness, I had to hope that Lucy would open up, talk about the past as a way to master it; sometimes the past trips patients up, sometimes it offers tools to handle new adversity.

No doctor ever gets a complete history from anyone. Why should I expect to? My patients are complicated, disguised, and contradictory. It is unclear who they are attacking and who they are resisting by their actions. For everything I heard from Lucy, it was clear there were ten things I didn't hear.

"The first time you were here, you told me that one of your goals was getting some productive work. Is that still the case?"

"I'd like to be working full-time so that I'm able to pay my bills with ease. Or in school of some kind, but I'd have to work part-time there, too. I can think of lots of work that I'd never do, like being a pharmaceutical company rep, for instance." She laughed. Even when she laughed, she didn't look me in the eye. "I have personal ethics. My family has values. My father has strong ideals about the world that he doesn't always apply to his life.

"Since I'll never get into graduate school because I was in college ten years ago, and I'll have to explain the black hole of my past, maybe I'll become a truck driver," she said teasingly. "I like to travel. I'd like to sleep in the back of a cab. I like to listen to music. I once hitchhiked from Boston to San Francisco. I'm happiest in a car or a train on a long trip. It still appeals to me."

"Why not be a truck driver then?" I asked, playing along.

"Besides for the fact that truck stops are filled with heroin and crack and crystal meth? Besides that it would let me fulfill my dream of being a functional drug addict?" She paused. "I never thought I'd end up really needing a job. I didn't, as juvenile as that sounds. I didn't think I'd be alive this long."

I took this in, but having already come to appreciate her intelligence and articulateness, I wanted to keep her looking toward the future. "What else would you like to have in a life without Vicodin?"

"I'd like to be happier than I am. Get more sleep. Feel less lonely. I'd like to have honest relations with people I feel connected to."

I had thought of Lucy as an addict from the first day I met her. As if being an addict was her sole identity. As if she was no longer a person who used Vicodin, but rather that Vicodin was a pre-condition for her being who she was. If she actually stopped using Vicodin, I wondered who she would be.

What I like about prescribing buprenorphine and caring for addicts is this: it is the beginning of something, a new life, a resto-ration. Most addicts are young, and so many of my older patients are waiting for bad news, or the end.

For just a second, Lucy stopped looking at the most distant corner of the ceiling and turned her full face to me. I was a little surprised to her see straight-on, her pretty mouth and thick dark hair, her red cheeks. It was like a gift.

PART II

CHAPTER 5

Monday, June 25

Peering into the waiting area of the clinic, I imagined the saddest circus on earth. Come see the greatest wheezer, the world's longest scar, the man who couldn't stop urinating, the most ravaged abdomen on seven continents, the woman who defecates into a bag. It was a freak show of plain-looking patients. On the TV, cantilevered from the ceiling in the corner, the announcer spoke about oil prices and the record tornado season in Oklahoma. I caught the name of a Middle Eastern country and saw footage of another young celebrity caught on film during some blasphemous loss of control. It was a rite of passage for recently famous movie stars, a stab at independence carried too far or too publicly. Every year four or five made the news for entering or leaving rehab—entering embarrassed, leaving repentant yet ready to a return to career and its privileges. It is difficult to believe the idea of addiction as a disease can hold much sway for the average viewer (or the clinic's patients-in-waiting) when the news depicts addiction as the starting up of drug use one notorious weekend and its end a few months later. What kind of disease can that be?

After her rocky first days of mixing her old pills with my new one, Lucy had done well, and our visits had become less frequent. It was now week eight. There had been no evidence of Vicodin in her last five urine tests, and she kept every appointment. I wrote her prescriptions by counting the number of pills she needed until her next visit. She ran out of her pills on the dates she was supposed to, suggesting she was taking the buprenorphine as prescribed, not selling it or sharing it or having it stolen by Brian.

I am into counting. With every patient, I count something— how many hours the effect of an inhaler will last, how many feet this one can walk before losing his breath, how long it takes that one to fall asleep, how many milligrams of nerve blocker are needed to relieve the tingling toes of another. Counting is scientific. Counting allows comparisons over time, a record, a means of organization, a defense against vagueness, forgetfulness, and chaos. When asking about alcohol use, my questions are, "How many drinking days have you had in the last month?" and "Were there ever days you had four or five drinks?" A casual drinker can safely enjoy one or two drinks a day. Is there such a thing as a casual Vicodin user? No user of nonprescribed opiates is respectable. Our cultural standard is that *any* unprescribed Vicodin is too much, even though Vicodin is not as unkind to the body as alcohol.

"How was South Carolina?" I asked Lucy. She had finally made it to Hilton Head the previous week, six weeks (and two canceled tickets) after her initial date.

"Four days is a long time to spend with my family even under the best of occasions. It's always depressing to see my parents. It shouldn't be. They're nice people. But I can't stand being around them."

She was wearing white corduroy pants and a crimson T-shirt, her black converse sneakers with pink laces. Her bright clothes contrasted with the no-color, no-fun coherence of my office, the aesthetic of decency. What is visible in my room is intended to make as little statement as possible. Should I have told Lucy that I didn't speak with my mother for a decade in the years following my father's death from heart failure at age sixty-four? Should I have shared with Lucy that my silence began with my mother leaving me, a fourteen-year-old, alone in a small suburban house on nights when she was on a date in the city twenty miles away? Should I have told her that when I was alone, I never had parties, never invited friends over to get drunk or high, but instead turned the television on loudly enough to cover noise of the house creaking until I fell asleep in the blue light? I'd taken my mother to live with me during the final eight years of her life when the dementia was evident and before lung cancer killed her. Our relationships with our parents can change.

Lucy's colorful clothes also contrasted with her mood. She gripped her white paper coffee cup, the tendons in her wrists strong. A tapestry shoulder bag lay across her lap, Nadine Gordimer's latest novel on top. Her head was turned as usual toward the door, and she adjusted herself sidewise in her regular seat.

"When did you get back?"

"Two days ago," Lucy answered. "This is why I can't stay clean."

It seemed as if she was telling me that she was using again, but something about her use of the present tense—"can't"—suggested the future tense to me—she was worried she would relapse, but

I sensed it hadn't happened in South Carolina. Her prognosis would have been poor if she'd started Vicodin again this early after beginning buprenorphine.

"Why can't you stay clean?"

"*This*. This is what always happens to me. I get miserable. I remember what a waste my life is. I visit my family and I don't know what to do. I feel like I don't belong in society. I hate lying to them about everything, little things, big things."

Her voice was lined with disgust and disappointment. She understood how uncertain her chances were.

Some patients enter my office and head straight for the examining table. They sit on the edge, fully clothed, feet dangling. They know the routine: a blood pressure check, a stethoscope slipped under a blouse toward the heart or applied to the back. I didn't need to examine Lucy today. What would I be looking or listening for? Yet checking her vital signs was an internist's duty and I stretched the blood pressure cuff to where she sat and banded it around her upper arm. When I pulled the black earpieces of the stethoscope away from my head and returned the inflatable device to its silver wall-mounted holder—the motions of normalcy—I asked, "What did you lie about?"

"There's no beginning or end to it. How much money I'm making, how happy I am."

"You feel you have to lie to them about the drugs?"

"They don't know what this year's been like at all."

"They must know more than you imagine."

"The number of things my mother has overlooked in my life is pathological. I almost can't believe the woman thinks I'm five years clean. She believes Brian ran through the $5,000 she gave me last year, and that I had nothing to do with it."

"Maybe you told her you've been clean for a while and gave

her reasons to blame your boyfriend. Maybe she takes you at your word?" I suggested.

I understood Lucy's complaints better than she imagined. Her mother expected her to lead a proper life, just as mine had of me: the career, the house, the spouse, the happiness, the respectability. Lucy had given her none of it. Outside, in the hall, I heard the shuffling of booted feet and coat snaps being popped open.

"I've lied, sure. But it doesn't really matter. She sums up the last fifteen years by trying to convince herself it hasn't been so bad. She lies to herself. She's always been determined not to believe me. Sometimes it's an uphill battle to convince her that I've used drugs at all. It doesn't matter what I did, or what I admit, she doesn't believe it. I'm not sure why she's never pieced things together."

I didn't accept that her mother really hadn't "pieced things together," but I was willing to play out the possibility for now. "Do you think she could have stopped your drug use if she had?"

Did Lucy want me to leave her alone? Did she want her prescription so she could get home? I ask questions because I believe, rightly or wrongly, that I can help a patient more completely if I have more information about them. I ask so many questions because I have absorbed the cultural belief that if a patient blathers on and the unconscious becomes conscious, it might make her better. I believe in catharsis. There is also clear evidence that talk therapy (a psychiatrist isn't required, an internist will do), combined with buprenorphine, produces less opiate relapse than buprenorphine alone. Indeed I've found that talking often exposes the risk of relapse, which might be discussed rather than acted on. In my office, conversation goes its own way, but I believe that asking patients to speak about difficult subjects lets them know themselves. It also lets me hear their longings and wishes, what they have lost, what terrifies them, how they believe their bodies and their loved ones have betrayed them.

"I blame her for being negligent, that's what it comes down to."

"Why do you think she was like that?"

"I don't know anything about her really. I know her mother was a horrible person. She died when I was twelve, but for ten years she'd been sick with diabetes, amputations, in nursing homes, babbling. I never knew her as anything but a sick person. And all I heard was that she was a horrible person. Even as a kid, I knew she was incapable of working. She was mean. She died at sixty. I guess she was crazy. She was on really heavy medications, I know that. Thorazine. She was really short—I don't know how I got so tall— with curly hair. She was Romanian, and had a younger sister, my great-aunt who was actually nice. I know my grandfather scared my father. My mother moved away with my father because she hated her father. She didn't hate her mother, but all she said about her when she died was, 'She tried. She did her best.' I remember once being taken out onto the porch by my grandfather who said, 'I don't know what you remember about your grandmother, but she was not a horrible woman.' I was sixteen. I remember because that summer he was sleeping on a foldout couch in the living room, and I was slipping in and out of the house in the warm weather to take acid with my oh-so-desirable friends. I was slipping out past him and slipping people in past him. Anyway, his comment tipped me off that she might have been a pretty difficult woman to be married to. But who knows?"

"You think your mother was negligent with you and your sister?"

"Not negligent. That's the wrong word, with this image of not giving us enough food. In some ways she was overly dutiful. What I mean is she was incapable of seeing what was before her eyes. On the other hand, I don't know what she could have done about me."

"And your father? Where is he in all this? What's he like?" I was waiting to hear the worst—that he beat her, sexually abused her, abandoned her. I was prepared to draw the arrow from the horrific violent father straight to the daughter's opiate addiction.

"Morose, embittered. A lawyer who hated everyone except his clients. Everyone he met, every lawyer he argued against, all my mother's friends. People were ignoramuses, or fascists. Those were his top two appraisals of people."

"Did he ever have a drug problem?"

"I'm sure he tried marijuana once when he was avoiding the draft. He's still into politics. He reads a lot. He thought I was a good writer in high school and wanted me to be a writer. He's got a temper. He always gets his way. He's hard to live with. He thinks my sister is spoiled; I'm his favorite."

"His favorite." I was surprised, although I tried not to sound it, so as not to offend her.

"One night when I was fifteen, I heard him and my mother throwing dishes in the kitchen. It was about ten o'clock, and I went downstairs to see what was going on and they told me that my drugs were causing the problem between them. My father screamed at me until four A.M. Then, all of a sudden, he was done screaming. The next day, I became his cause. He was going to save me. My father, the man who had been wronged by everyone, was going to do whatever he had to do to save me. And it's been like that ever since."

"So it sounds like they all knew about your drug use."

"My dad did. Every time I stayed out overnight during high school, he'd go to the police and declare me missing. He was on a crusade and I avoided him. I was using, so you could say

I didn't want to see my parents because I was ashamed. Or that I just wanted to use and didn't want interference from anyone. After I left for college, which they paid for, I barely spoke to them again.

"All I know is that my mother still goes on the theory that I have some sort of problem, but my boyfriends are always more of the problem, and I've been the unwitting victim. Please. Give me a little credit. As if I don't know how to get myself in trouble? She just thinks I need to get out of whatever relationship I'm in, and she's not wrong. Maybe she does believe what I tell her now. I can't believe anyone believes me anymore. What if I told her that I love drugs more than her? She wouldn't believe that. That won't fly. Does it really matter what she knows about my life at this time?"

I am not a pure behaviorist who somehow believes that patients, years into an addiction, can be trained in a matter of weeks out of urges and cravings, that they can be taught to force the mind always toward better, more productive thoughts, which allows one to not deal with the past. I believe buprenorphine literally gives patients the chance to change their minds about whether to continue to use narcotics, and without medication it is almost impossible for an opiate addict to get her bearings. But medication isn't enough. I am not a psychiatrist, but I want my patients to feel attended to; I want to give them the chance to size me up and decide it is worth the risk to share their troubles with me, and that takes more time. Some days I need to keep the visit brief because I know I have patients who will require longer appointments coming later in the day. But some days a patient begins speaking, and she isn't really speaking to me, but to herself, and it isn't what she intended to say, but there it is, audible, and a surprise to the both of us, and I never would have heard the story if I hadn't handed over an extra twenty or thirty minutes.

Lucy, on the days when she felt like talking, was good company.

"Which part of your life during the past year do you think would be most upsetting to your mother if you told the truth?" I asked.

"That I'm alone ninety percent of the time, not doing anything. That I don't know anyone. I've lived my whole life in this town and the only people I know anymore are drug addicts. The only people who talk to me are people on the street who ask me for money or ask me where Brian is so they can get high with him. That I quit my job and have no savings."

Was she alone (and if so, where was Brian?) or did she *feel* alone? I didn't interrupt.

"I'm afraid to talk to people, to ask for help. I don't know why I'm afraid, I just am. Everyone looks happy to me. I can't stop drugs without getting depressed. I sat inside in South Carolina for four days crying. I'm not going to a psychiatrist, either, so don't ask," she commanded.

At 9:30 A.M. my room was illuminated by the spare light of early New England spring. What was she staring at on the back of my office door? What did she see in the wood grain—a topographical map, mittens, vines, silhouettes of celebrities?

It is not uncommon to hear a patient say that she is depressed. But depression means many things to patients. They report being depressed when they don't know what to do with themselves, have periods of sadness, can't sit still, are restless or sleepless or irritable. They might call themselves depressed if they feel down for even four days, even if the particular four days were spent in South Carolina around family they hadn't seen in over two years. I wasn't sure if Lucy was suffering from depression. But I knew that if I sent her to a colleague of mine who was a psychiatrist, he would say, "I can't tell you if your patient is depressed until she stops using Vicodin. Have her get clean for at least three months and then come to see me." To make a depression diagnosis, my consulting psychiatrist would have wanted to check off a list of symptoms in order to ascertain that Lucy had experienced a majority of them consistently over weeks. But the symptoms of opiate dependence and depression overlap.

Every research study done in the past two decades has determined that more than half of all narcotic addicts had a history of diagnosable, persistent depression at some point in their lives. This may have been due to the long-term depressive effects of drugs, or to a shared genetic liability of depression and drug dependence—people with a particular brain chemistry who were likely to get addicted to opiates were also likely to get depressed. But was Lucy depressed now? Depressed enough to require an antidepressant medication in addition to the buprenorphine? Calling herself depressed was one thing, but was it important to make a diagnosis, assign her another diagnostic label and start another medication immediately in order to improve her mood, her life, her risk of returning to Vicodin?

Addicts often find that narcotics serve as antidepressants, as medications to control their moods. Vicodin offers a form of relief, as Julia and many others who see the world as unaccommodating and harsh have reported. Vicodin reduced the stresses of life for Julia and made her feel "superhuman." Vicodin is armor, a way of comforting oneself. It is a way to get away from painful feelings, from the burden of human contact, the inability to accomplish enough on any given day, the dark pressure of private thoughts. I believe patients when they tell me that narcotics help improve their mood, although I wonder if someone using Vicodin, OxyContin, or heroin daily has an accurate perception of their energy level, their feelings of peace. Still, in America of 2009, opiates are not FDA approved to treat anxiety or depression, and no mainstream (and self-protective) doctor prescribes them for mood disorders. In the end, Vicodin is a lousy antidepressant, as Julia learned: it requires escalating doses, and taken secretly, produces guilt during unchecked use.

With Julia, who always forced her beautiful Mona Lisa smile when she came in, it was unclear if she was more depressed or anxious. At her first visit, Julia had talked about "staying calm" on Vicodin. But after months on buprenorphine, her mood was worse. She felt fine during the day but had a difficult transition to home, where she was jittery and unfocused. After a day at the office, there were too many things waiting to get done at home. She found managing housework difficult. She used to enjoy making dinner but didn't anymore. She didn't like cleaning up, or preparing the next day's lunch for her children, or bathtime with the two girls she hadn't seen all day. At the same time, she admitted to having palpitations. Her heart was racing and her mind was, too. She told me, "I don't have much to worry about. Not more than most people. But everyone else seems to handle it easily." She felt guilty that it was left to her husband to pull things together. "He's dealing with all of it. It's so unfair to him when all I want is to watch TV or lay in bed for an entire weekend day. He never just collapses on the couch. I wish he would. But he wants to help and goes right to it when he sees that I can't." I thought that her husband must have been furious with her, or confused, but she didn't speak much about him.

Just after she'd started buprenorphine, she'd been out to dinner with friends, women she hadn't seen much of during the past year because she didn't want them to pick up on her Vicodin use. The meal hadn't gone well. "During dinner I had this urge to get up and leave. They had a lot of questions for me. They knew I had been going through something. I told them I was having a tough time with an ill family member, which was true, my sister's very sick. I didn't get into other stuff; I don't ever want to. They weren't letting it rest, though. They wanted details. I'm good at changing the subject, but their questions were exactly why I hadn't seen them in a year. I felt claustrophobic. I couldn't breathe. I wanted to leave. I really felt that I couldn't continue sitting at the table. But I let it ride out. It lasted about fifteen minutes.

"By the end of dinner, my friends thought I was on tons of antidepressants. Together, they had come up with this theory. They kept joking, 'How many therapists are you seeing? Who turned you around?' One said, 'I wish I could speak to someone, too.' I said, 'You should. It does wonders.' I played along that they had the right diagnosis."

Depression was acceptable for Julia, announceable, but not substance abuse. Depression wasn't a person's fault; addiction was.

"On the drive home, I thought about how, in the past year, I've been anxious whenever I was out with people, and how I didn't go out much. When I went, I really didn't participate in the conversation. I took extra pills to control my nerves before I went to any family occasion."

The vulnerability to addiction is always emotional (and in retrospect can generally be discerned before the substance became available). Julia described panic attacks, but also days sunk in bed under the covers. I wondered whether the buprenorphine had uncovered a deep history of anxiety, or whether her distress at dinner with her friends was only the fear of discovery. I wondered whether she was depressed or if her symptoms were a matter of suffering from the effects of feeling terribly guilty and not being honest with her husband.

"What if your friends knew what was really going on with you?" I asked Julia.

"I don't know. I'd never want them to," she answered. "I think one had an idea, though. About three months ago, she didn't ask me directly, but she said to me, 'If I didn't know you better, I'd think you were taking drugs. But I know you so well.'

"I can't stop thinking about how I could have prevented all this; but if I think about it too much, I don't want to do anything."

Were her low moods and nervousness more apparent three months into treatment because Vicodin had been better at ameliorating her depressive and anxiety symptoms than buprenorphine? Or was she feeling worse because now she was looking at her life differently, without the pursuit of drugs? Julia had emerged from a year of opiate use without serious health, career, or financial effects. She hadn't ruined her life, but life had changed, not only during her year of use, but now, and forever.

With Lucy Fields, who had lurched from one drug to another during her early twenties, I knew it would be nearly impossible to untangle her moods from her addictions. She couldn't describe how she functioned *before* she started using drugs because there hadn't been such a period as an adult. I knew I would have to ask about her family to know if any of her close relatives suffered from depression. It seemed quite likely that she was depressed in addition to being addicted to Vicodin; she could have both together. Addicts frequently have multiple problems; it is rare to find an alcoholic or narcotic addict who doesn't also have anxiety, depression, an eating disorder, or another manner of self-harming behavior.

When I start addicts on buprenorphine, replacing out-of-control use of narcotics with my own once-a-day controlled prescription, I am equally likely to see one of three results: about a third report they are no longer "depressed"; a third said they don't notice any change in mood; and the final third feel worse. That the moods of many addicts dramatically improve within weeks of starting buprenorphine indicates to me that opiates themselves are not the cause of depression, because chemically buprenorphine is almost identical to the abusable opiates. Rather, some addicts probably improve because they no longer fear being arrested or found out by their spouse, or are no longer worried about emptying their bank accounts to find the next day's stash. As a patient said to me not long ago, "I was depressed because I wasn't doing the right thing. The better I do, the better I feel."

But a good number of my patients become more depressed after starting buprenorphine. Life seems stale, colorless, slow, and dull without drugs. Quitting often brings a sense of panic and doom. The addict at first thinks pessimistically about the future. "I'll never be able to sleep well or relax or have enough energy to work a full day. I've given up my peace and solace." In addition, looking around, a patient might finally realize he has no car, no income. He is ashamed, embarrassed. Recognizing a bad situation, his dignity erodes. And whose fault is it? His own, he knows. For starting in the first place, and now for stopping. He is depressed in my office, but I wonder if he was depressed before he started (Vicodin as antidepressant) or only after he stopped. Is Vicodin treatment or cause or both?

Recently, a woman addicted to heroin came in asking to start an antidepressant. I asked her to think about giving up her heroin, but she didn't want to—she said it was the only medication that controlled her back pain. Karen was heavily made up, with brown hair streaked blond, and she wore high-heeled red leather boots. She was willing to buy the heroin, but she wanted me to provide (and her insurance company to pay for) a medication for her low mood. She probably was depressed, but I wasn't certain. She had only recently started taking heroin again two months ago, after a three-year hiatus, and just before that, she had been withdrawn and disinterested in her realty work; she sounded depressed even talking about those years. I decided to give her a medication, hoping it would serve as a foundation for quitting heroin again. I chose not to tell her right then that I fundamentally didn't believe she could continue using narcotics and feel better. I chose not to tell her my belief that the heroin would likely mask the benefit of any antidepressant. But I did tell her her life would be better without heroin, no matter what medication I offered.

Lucy didn't want to see a psychiatrist and she didn't want an antidepressant medication ("I don't have any faith in what it will do. I don't know a way to relax except Vicodin. I should get a Vicodin script for life because I need it," she half-joked). She wanted to stop Vicodin, but without it, she felt she was just a woman without money in the bank whose boyfriend was an addict, a woman interested in independence, but young and scared.

Did she sit inside weeping in South Carolina because she saw her life clearly, or because she believed she'd lost access to the feeling of real emotion she still believed Vicodin afforded her after a decade? In withdrawal, her pain had been physical; she'd focused on that. Was her weeping an expression of her regret about the decision to quit Vicodin, or the beginning of finding a way to address mental discomfort?

"Tell me about your parents' place down there."

"They live in your basic Hilton Head gated community. Identical tan and white two-story houses ringing an artificial pond. Duck shit covering the Bermuda grass going down to the water. Lots of sliding glass doors and sprinkler systems. Corrugated gray sheet metal sunblocks over the cars in the driveway. No one under sixty in sight."

"Did you get out of the house at all?"

"She took me bird-watching. My mother likes birds. She's

pretty good at spotting them, too. She doesn't really have friends there. She'd probably have more if it weren't for my father. She's fairly nice, but even in retirement he finds a reason to dislike everyone. We have cousins who live nearby who want to befriend her, but he doesn't want them around. He's miserable. He's a step beyond passively not liking people—he doesn't want to see anyone. He's had a couple of friends his whole life. Nobody meets his high standards. He does seem to understand the depths of misery, even my misery, but our connection on that level is brief. His siblings all hate each other, his father was mentally ill. The family's a mess. Sometimes he's loving to me, but more often he's angry; he insults, swears. You can't go near him. My mother tolerates him, pacifies him. I dread going home because I never know his mood." She held her neck, closed her eyes, and took a deep breath.

I wondered if her father was depressed, if he'd ever been treated.

"What else did you do down there?"

She looked up at me briefly. She knew I was asking whether she had used any Vicodin in South Carolina.

"I took my buprenorphine every day. Every morning, right before my coffee. It ruins the flavor, you know."

"I've heard that from a few other people." I smiled to let her know that she hadn't really told me yet what I needed to know and I was about to ask her outright. "No drug use when you were away?"

Some addicts talk nonstop about drugs when they aren't using, like a dieter talks about nothing but food when she is trying to lose weight. It is a way of keeping the taste in your mouth. Lucy hadn't yet spoken about drugs today.

During these early weeks of sobriety, when the risk of relapse is highest, the peril is rarely acknowledged. Patient and doctor want to believe it will never happen. But relapse is a real contingency that can be worked against and beaten, although not by pretending it doesn't exist. To talk about the possibility of restarting Vicodin is going to be a part of every visit with me. An addict's promise never to use again is ironclad until it isn't. I knew and Lucy knew it wasn't, so what was the point of being cagey? In every attempt to quit there was a proviso on page 3, paragraph 1 of the make-believe contract, "*Unless I want to use again.*"

"I had no drugs to use in South Carolina," Lucy said. "I actually went to an NA meeting. I found one in the newspaper. Of course my parents didn't let me drive the car, even though I've never crashed one of theirs. But no one is allowed to drive my father's car. He's very territorial. He won't let my mother drive it."

Narcotics Anonymous is a peer-directed, self-governing, abstinence-goaled, spiritual program of twelve steps. Recovering addicts stand up in front of other addicts, and share their experiences, losses, and pledges, as the audience in the church basement or hospital cafeteria listen hard, drinking coffee and smoking cigarettes. In America, if addicts walked out their front door looking for help, half the time they end up at an NA or AA meeting, far more often than they go to mental health specialists or doctors.

"They've never been willing to take me to any support group meetings," Lucy added. "It's not that my mother disapproves. She just doesn't want me to identify myself as an addict my whole life. My mother would rather I go to a support group for the mentally ill. She thinks I should see a psychiatrist. There is substantial mental illness in my family, no drugs though."

That Lucy's mother preferred to think her daughter was mentally ill rather than an addict told me she knew more about Lucy's history than I had originally thought, and that she ranked her daughter's problems in a hierarchy of bad news that most Americans would support. Every parent, if forced to choose, wants their son or daughter to have a psychiatric disorder—which more and more are believed to be treatable—rather than an addiction. Perhaps only schizophrenia seems more damaging and personally painful than substance abuse.

"I thought I should try a meeting. I've been to a few over the past ten years.

"On the bus ride over, there were two people behind me who were going to the meeting. It was as if Brian had followed me to South Carolina and was talking to one of his scumbag friends, that's how familiar it was as I was listening to them. I was thinking I have more in common with them than I do with anyone in my family. They were talking about friends in prison and the fire they set in their apartment. They were hatching some intricate detox scheme. That's who's hanging around Brian at our apartment these days."

I had one picture of Lucy's current life with Brian, but I was starting to get another. It sounded rougher, harsher than I'd originally thought. I had a picture of her quietly taking her Vicodin pills and retreating to her room to listen to music or watch a movie. I thought of Brian as a sometimes-intrusive roommate who shared an interest with her in narcotics but he had his own tough circle, too. I wondered if he hit her, threatened her.

"I've never liked meetings. Too many creepy old men. Meetings are creepy and religious, and they promote not-thinking."

I'd been to NA meetings as an observer over the years to check out the scene. The group was always a little tense at first in the squinty light. Then an old-timer with lousy teeth and long months of sobriety under his belt stood and started his story, got a laugh over his announcement of some misery everyone could relate to (some totally justified ass-kicking by wife, boss, or mother), and then the group relaxed. I could imagine Lucy in the back row, sitting sideways in her chair, self-conscious and keeping her head down.

"I went because I had nowhere else to go," she said. "I had to push myself to go. I had to get out of the house and where else was there? Who goes to meetings? People with no support who feel unwanted. I always feel alienated at meetings. I should be getting the opposite feeling, sympathy, empathy, something. But then I think: If I don't belong at meetings, where do I belong? I can identify on one level, but I'm from a different world, going back to my parents' gated condo as soon as I'm done there. I can't hang out with street people. I don't want to share my story. They give you the same lines over and over. *Put God first.* They're like evangelists. That bothers me. When someone says, 'The hand of God lifted you out of the gutter,' that's just really weird. Don't you think that's weird?"

She laughed and I had to laugh with her.

"I can't force myself to share. I don't want to share. I just don't. I don't. What the hell is there to tell? Where do I start? Maybe I don't believe in the value of spilling my guts to a room of people." She knew it was heretical to bad-mouth the meeting. Still, she didn't like the exhortation and she didn't identify with the speakers.

NA's reputed success is easy to cast aside: those who go to meetings are more serious about quitting drugs, and might succeed without attending NA meetings. But what if you took a hundred addicts and assigned fifty to go to meetings, obliged them to go as part of addiction care even if they didn't want to go. Would they do better than the fifty who were not mandated? In one study, they did.

NA isn't merely a place for the lonely to go looking for a group of strangers who are willing to give you a pat on the back. The meetings offer a way to handle stress—NA philosophy suggests it is good to call friends and make plans as a way to cope. More important, for people without friends or whose only friends use opiates, it offers a ready-made group who can be trusted to listen, and better yet, support one's abstinence. If an addict meets people who have successfully quit, he or she can become more motivated to quit. It is this personal involvement with NA, accepting fellowship from and doing services for others in the group, that is more important than the number of meetings an addict attends. I suggest at least one visit to NA to every patient with a narcotic addiction, but many still don't take me up on it.

Lucy went to the meeting in South Carolina to get a break from her parents, but she wasn't likely to go back from what I'd just heard. She wasn't interested in a spiritual awakening in a church basement. "I don't want to share my story," she'd said. And she wasn't alone. Contrary to stereotype, the most common reason women give for not going to NA or AA meetings is not wanting to stand up in front of a group and talk about their feelings. I didn't yet have a clear view of how Lucy was doing this month, but I appreciated her honesty and her skepticism and her go-it-alone detachment. I wasn't a joiner, either.

Patients who made the effort to go to NA meetings valued plenty of things about the meetings beside the free cookies and coffee. They liked comparing stories of psychic pain and mounting losses, of the worst things they'd done while using. They liked retelling tales of their attempts to taper off drugs and their longest binges. There was always someone who had it worse. They'd lost professions and keys to the house and every single friend and any chance of having fun. They'd picked up phobias and dreads, headaches, long histories of stays in rehab and detox and persistent fears of insanity. Speaking the words offered a kind of integrity, a link to the world. For one hour, part of life still seemed intact. They didn't come expecting to be thanked for their stories, but they appreciated the gratitude nonetheless.

Addicts tell me that being at a meeting was like attending a reunion with people they'd already seen in the mirror. They wanted to be around people who knew it wasn't easy to quit. People who had asked themselves the unanswerable question: if I want to quit, why can't I? They wanted a simple answer to that one, but knew it wasn't forthcoming. Inside the meeting, everyone was a seeker. They wanted to know it was possible to succeed, to lick this thing for good, to quit for all time. They wanted to believe that things could change.

They also wanted to be consoled. If they told their stories outside this basement they would sound whiney and self-absorbed and self-pitying and pathetic. But here, there was an acceptance of the everyday struggles with little things, with shopping and cooking and being good to your kids. They didn't come thinking they were unique. They wanted their guilt and self-disgust mitigated through sharing the stories of serious trouble. They wanted to study the crowd and see looks not of concern, but familiarity.

Most of my buprenorphine patients refuse to go to NA, and they click their tongues at me when I even suggest the idea. Marco went to a meeting at my insistence and told me, "I don't like the war stories. I don't want to hear about people running around crazy. I don't like the people. I always worked for money. I never stole. When they describe their time out there, I'm so turned off. I'm not out there robbing. I want a meeting with working people more like me, you know what I mean? You have to do what works for you and that meeting didn't work for me."

Many patients who have gone were afraid they would run into

someone they knew. They also didn't want to be around other addicts. They wanted to help themselves, or get a little support from me, in the privacy of this office. They didn't like the vocabulary of sin and redemption. If addiction was enthrallment to a false god, they didn't want to be led to the truth.

But sometimes they asked themselves what they had to lose by going? They had no faith in themselves anymore. Their judgment was questionable.

None of the twelve steps involves buprenorphine. My patient Tom had been told by an NA group that taking buprenorphine was simply replacing one drug with another. No matter what your doctor claimed, you were still manacled (methadone, too, was called liquid handcuffs). Tom went to a meeting and it was clear that he was not welcome back if he was using any medication. But I've also heard that from meeting to meeting there is no consensus on this point. Some meetings are unwilling to punish addicts for regaining their lives in whatever way they possibly can.

"I can't stand meetings. I can't take them," Lucy said. "I can't take the listening. I hate the higher power shit. The 'on your knees and pray' shit.

"But if I don't go to meetings, I feel like I'm missing out on something," she said guiltily. "I feel like I'm missing the bonding, supportive environment. I'm not sure how much of that is even true and how much is propaganda. Meetings have never been exactly warm and inviting to me. I guess I could meet decent people there, but everyone Brian meets at a meeting he ends up buying from or using with."

"But it was a relief to get out of the house," I suggested.

"Except that I'm a magnet for older, predatory men. When I got there, all the creepy men came up to me, an under-thirty female visitor, someone they'd never seen before. It's a real problem for women. It's why, if I ever go to another meeting, I'd prefer a women-only group if I could ever find one. The men just surrounded me and asked if I needed anything: cigarettes, money, a ride."

She sounded annoyed, but also a tiny bit amused and flattered by the attention.

"*Did* you need a ride?"

"My mother actually picked me up. Somehow she got my father to release the car. When I got in next to her, she asked me, 'What the hell was that? A circle of men around you?'"

Lucy laughed. Her pink shoelaces bounced. "Six men and me must have been quite a sight for her. My mother used to scream at me, 'Are you stupid?' when she saw the men who came to pick me up in the past. Of course she let me date them, men ten years older."

She was silent for a moment.

"She says she's not ashamed of me, but I know she is."

"It's hard to see your parents because it feels like you've let them down," I offered.

"This is beyond letting them down. Not getting into Yale was letting them down. What I've done with my life is unfathomable. No wonder my mother can't admit to my history. She has no context to put it in.

"The time when I was living with them is long over. Who am I to complain? I don't know. Part of me wants to forget about it all. If I could use drugs today and forget about everything from back then, I would. You hear addicts say all the time, 'I started using to have fun,' but that was never true for me. I never used to have a good time—maybe there was an element of not wanting to fit in, or I thought it would automatically get me friends—but I didn't use to have a good time. I mean the first time I ever drank,

I blacked out and woke up to find some guy groping me, and then I threw up eight times. I was after some kind of forgetting. I wanted to push the world aside. I guess there were some times it made me happy for a while. But I had such disgust and revulsion for myself. I let men do whatever they wanted to me."

She stopped herself. Again, she wasn't ready to tell me more.

Interviews are complicated. There are places where the conversation goes and places it doesn't go. Lucy's telling had a choppy forward motion. But she was not speaking to me to gain self-knowledge. She was unsure about the value of introspection. Here she was, unharmed and recognizable, having survived a hard time. She talked to convince herself that all was not lost.

I looked through the thick glass of my sealed office window (you can lean hard against it without fear of falling) where pollen on the outside blurred the lower edge of my view. On the narrow, cluttered, busy street, ambulances pressed in toward the hospital's sliding doors. After dark, this scene would be just as filled and active. I liked the dense packing of sickness—all in one place—of the emergency department. Stretchers lowered and lifted, and were conducted inside with decorum. Into the physician's territory. One had to seek permission to enter one of the stripped-down cubicles of that place. The ED doctor's charm was brief, his hospitality unlasting. A patient came in and he saw them out, just as he'd let others out for years. The emergency room doctor's job was to stabilize and transfer. What was mine, after the diagnosis? At least to treat, which included listening for as long as it took.

"I didn't speak this much the whole time I was in South Carolina." She didn't need to be interrogated—she did that to herself.

Over the years, I imagined, in the warfare between parent and child, Lucy had been resentful and ugly, angry and self-destructive. She must have assumed her mother had never forgiven her; she had never forgiven herself. I still didn't understand why she'd decided to visit her parents after not seeing them for years.

"It sounds like a tough visit. Did any of it make you *want* to use?"

"I don't need a visit to my parents to make me want to use."

I didn't think Lucy had used narcotics in South Carolina. I stood and walked to the cabinet over the sink, pulled on the cold metal handle, reached into the middle of three neatly organized shelves, and withdrew a plastic cup and a clear plastic bag. I handed both to her.

The toxicology results would confirm whether she'd used in the past three days, which was how long narcotics or their metabolites hung around in the body. I had no test that would inform me about what she'd taken further back.

As always, handing her the cup implied, without uttering a word, "I don't trust you; prove it to me," although I did trust her today.

She took the supplies and left my office, heading down the hall to the bathroom. Worried they will be expelled from care, many addicts learn how to hide evidence of recent drug use. Toxicological testing has become a technological race. When I was working with Lucy, our medical laboratory tested urine for body temperature (to confirm its recent provision and that it was not hidden under a parka and brought in cold, collected on another day when they hadn't used), and for chemistry (to confirm this was in fact urine and not apple juice). There were also test-cups that could give nearly instantaneous results, but they were expensive and my clinic required me to submit specimens to a central laboratory. I would have the results by the end of the day.

Even though the visit had started by Lucy telling me it had been "depressing" to see her parents, even though she said she'd spent days weeping and left the Hilton Head house only twice during a long weekend, I never thought she was deeply depressed. She'd arrived promptly, had interacted, and smiled and laughed during our conversation. She was too talkative and peaceful for me to be alarmed about her mental state.

Even if her urine showed signs of narcotic use, I wouldn't discharge her from treatment. I thought about how often I spoke to patients in the negative, punishing language of medicine. "You haven't lost enough weight," "You didn't respond to antibiotics," "You failed chemotherapy." I had gotten into the habit of calling positive toxicology results "dirty" urines. This implied the addict herself was dirty—she was trash, garbage, unsanitary. The urine of the drug-free addict was "clean." She had not polluted her bloodstream. Vicodin was a tyrant; did I have to be one also with my vocabulary of clean and dirty?

As I thought about the day's visit with Lucy, I realized that to enjoy treating addicts (because if you didn't enjoy it, you wouldn't last), one needed a sense of irony, the belief that everyone's life vacillated between euphoria and sorrow, and an acceptance that this group of patients would likely be too self-involved ever to be grateful. In all my years, only one addict, Joe, has ever said thank you. He told me I was a "good guy" for "sticking with him during hard times." He had just gotten a job as a handyman after six months wondering if he could pay the bills, asking his grown sons, for the first time, to contribute to the house expenses. He'd lost his health insurance, but I hadn't deserted him. He didn't have cash and I'd given him a free pass on visit costs. He did offer to barter labor ("I'm really a good tiler, you should come see my work someday"). Although he hated handouts, I'd even gotten him free buprenorphine from the company that manufactured it. Joe didn't like being in debt and he got out of it by being thankful, and months later referring a friend of his to me.

Lucy returned to the room with her urine cup in the bag. She handed it to me and moved toward her chair. The left back pocket of her jeans was torn off.

"When I left for South Carolina, Brian told me he was going to stop using, too. But he kept calling when I was down there, like ten times a day, and when I finally called back from Hilton Head, I knew he was using. It was obvious. At least to me.

"When I got back, he wasn't at the airport to pick me up. I knew exactly what was going on. He was out of his mind when I'd spoken to him on the phone. He was getting high with money I'd left. He's a bad liar. I'd know what to look for, don't you think? He was in the hospital with broken ribs. He'd crashed the car he'd borrowed. He's known for rolling cars. He's had more than one DUI. He is constantly nodding at the wheel even when he isn't high. He's just a bad driver. Brian is the worst driver I've ever seen even when he isn't on narcotics. Plus, he has no license. He's destroyed every car he ever had. He hurt people, including himself.

"I called him on the cell phone. 'I'm in the hospital,' he said. 'Someone came up behind me and drove me off the road. I broke six ribs.' I didn't really care at that point. He'd driven into a tree. They had to take him out with the jaws of life.

"'This is it,' I told him. 'I'm not coming home. I'm getting my stuff and leaving.' 'You selfish bitch. I'm in the hospital,' he said. 'You'll live,' I told him. I didn't feel that guilty saying it. I hate him. He said he wanted to quit, but of the two of us, I had greater resolution, as all the evidence shows.

"When he didn't show up at the airport, I had a feeling of relief. I called my friend Sean and he picked me up. He took me to my apartment. It smelled like cat shit, and there were syringes and cottons and needles everywhere. Brian had been shooting up. The place was disgusting. I'd been living with it, but that day, I couldn't stand it. I took one bag of clothes. 'Don't you want to take your stuff?' Sean asked me. 'What about all your furniture?' He had a van. I just wanted to get out."

When she'd spoken about Brian before, none of it was flattering or affectionate. Based on the little I knew, I had imagined that she lived with Brian in harsh conditions, with few belongings in tiny oppressive rooms. The kind of apartment that made you eager to be outside in the fresh, vast air.

"I had no interest in being with Brian even before I went away."

Now I understood why she'd gone to Hilton Head. Not to rekindle good feelings toward her parents, but to get away from Brian. She couldn't have known he would flip a car, but she must have hoped he'd do something that would convince her finally to put an end to their relationship.

"I don't even like him really," Lucy said. "He was just a using partner for eighteen months."

"He was using heroin?"

"Over the past ten months. He said it was cheaper than the Vicodin and OxyContin he'd used before. First he snorted the heroin, then he started injecting."

"Where'd you meet him?" I asked.

"Ironically, I met him at a bar. I was living at my parents' in Attleboro just before they moved to Hilton Head."

"What was his attraction?"

"We started seeing each other and he would bring me candy—lollipops, Swedish fish, gummy bears. I ate candy everywhere and he immediately picked up on that. I can't believe I have a tooth left.

"I had no apartment, no job, no money, no way to leave my parents' house. He had an apartment, and he wasn't using. I knew, even from the first relatively normal dates that he wouldn't stay clean. I was on and off Vicodin because I couldn't afford it. He said I seemed miserable. He didn't seem to have bad motives, I thought. He said on our third date that I was so miserable, he was becoming miserable. He turned it into a game. We'll get high and you'll feel better, he'd say. One day he got me about twenty Vicodins, and he had to use, too, of course. I had my 'medicine,' he said, and he had to take some medicine to be able to live with me. The next day he bought himself heroin, which I'd never tried, but which he'd used for years on and off. Was I attracted to him? No. But my whole life, if you were attracted to me, I'd go along. I had a million times before. At least he wasn't violent."

Unlike heroin, pills such as Vicodin, FDA approved for pain relief, at least have a factory-made certainty about them (although fakes are peddled rampantly on the Internet). Heroin buyers are unsure of what they are getting. Heroin is often cut with inert ingredients—baking soda, talc, sugar, laundry detergent. The percentage of pure opiate varies by day, neighborhood, dealer. Quality matters to addicts, but when withdrawal symptoms begin, only price matters.

"When I called him in the hospital to tell him I'd moved out, he was so pathetic. 'I can't live without you. I'll kill myself. I'll get clean. I love you so much.' He gave me that whole routine. I thought briefly of going back. He was manipulative and I felt guilty. But for eighteen months we'd been sitting in a room, using drugs, not seeing anyone else. Enough was enough.

"I can really pick them. Brian was pathetic. Mark, before him? He was much worse. He was an addict, too, but violent, murderously violent toward women."

No matter what her toxicology results showed when they came back today, no matter what had happened with Mark, Brian, or her parents in the past, my relationship with Lucy, and her new relationship to drugs, was defined solely by what happened between the two of us in this room. All that mattered now was that she had a sense that *I* had some sense of how hard all this was for her. There probably hadn't been a lot of people who'd been nice to her recently. The more I learned of her life, the more it seemed unbearable to me, filled with threats and tedium and sorrow. Sorrow shapes many patients, and sorrow connects them to their doctors. (Opiates poison sorrow, one of its favorable qualities.) I am a great protector of sad memories and I carry my own, which I visit regularly. I am a champion of sorrowful moments; I believe that properly examined, opened up and touched, they bring not only a private peace, but also protection, a kind of melancholy good luck.

"Did you ever try some of his heroin?" I expected a sanitized report.

"I did. A few times."

This didn't surprise me. Few addicts try one form of opiate and stick with it alone. In her youth, Lucy had experimented, moving from alcohol to cough syrup to hallucinogens and finally narcotics, dabbling in marijuana along the way. Cigarettes were a continuous attraction, yet at the first visit she had not admitted to anything other than narcotics—she didn't use Valium, cocaine, or any of the newer club drugs like ecstasy. She also hadn't admitted to other examples of lost control common to drug users. She wasn't bulimic. She didn't cut herself. She didn't go to the track or casinos.

That she had tried heroin with her boyfriend was not unusual. Having a drug-using companion meant she didn't have to hide her pills from at least one person. She already concealed her drug life from parents, employers, the outside world. She didn't have to be discreet about opiates around Brian, and she could use as much as she wanted. She didn't blame Brian for her use of heroin or anything else. It was too easy to think of her as a victim, with a man as the villain. She put herself in the path of heroin and it had appeared. She made herself an easy target.

I had the sense that even when addicts use together—sharing drugs or paraphernalia—they are essentially using alone. From Lucy's description of the people who hung around her apartment, there was little eye contact, laughter, or genuine conversation. Each user concentrated on how the drug made him or her feel. I wondered if this was what she meant when she told me she was alone 90 percent of the time.

Is there something worse about heroin than Vicodin? Although the common image of a heroin user is a destitute, urban male, Vicodin users do no better quitting their opiate habit than heroin injectors. Heroin has a certain lingering glamour (*Pulp Fiction*) as well as a darker cultural stigma. Heroin injection is a throwback nowadays; the purity of heroin on the streets is such that sniffing, a safer and less complicated procedure, provides nearly as good a high. Aficionados still claim that injection, with its direct and rapid delivery, is unmatchable, but there are nasty risks to needle use—physical and legal—and the cost of equipment, the mess of carrying and cleaning one's "kit," makes it less attractive to many opiate users. Heroin and Vicodin users have equally high risk of dropout from my buprenorphine program. The pharmacology is a little different—the heroin addict uses four times a day if he or she can afford it, the Vicodin user two or three times a day—but every opiate addict starts to feel a low-level discomfort at a certain hour and to still it, only more opiate does the trick, and then the whole pharmacological cycle starts up again.

Heroin users talk about getting high more than do Vicodin

addicts. Whenever I have *asked* a heroin addict what it was like to get high, they always looked annoyed. Among all my questions, this one was almost unacceptable. At first I thought the irritation came from not being able to remember the high. Then I believed their impatience was due to the question being too private. I was intruding. But finally I discovered the shared belief that almost any discussion about getting high diminished the experience or the memory somehow. It was as if the vast and rich and blurry sensation they had had, and would have again if they were lucky, the head rush and the body's disappearance, would be harmed by speech. I have never heard anything negative from an active heroin user who had no interest in quitting: getting high was a tall experience that threw a very short shadow. According to addicts, it is unlike cocaine, which makes you jittery and tense. It is unlike Valium, which makes you spacey and sluggish. A heroin high contains many separate and diverse feelings, not one. Heroin is a warm fog, monochromatic and gray, serene and enclosing. A flash of numbness, followed by contentment. Relaxation—the way crying with delight relaxes you. A feeling of seeing things from a different angle, free from the claims of aging, caution, fear. Time is gone; clocks stopped; deadlines expired. Now and forever combined.

Had Lucy used a lot or a little heroin with Brian? A few times, or for a few months? Was she underplaying her heroin use? I was suspicious. At our first appointment I'd asked her about heroin and she had denied even trying it.

"I only used with Brian." Heroin has a mystique, a certain coolness that might have appealed to her. But more likely it was just what was around and she wanted to try something new.

"Did you inject it?" I asked.

"Only twice. I don't like needles."

"Why did you stop?"

"You really want to know? I associated heroin with the time when I started doing bad stuff. We robbed people. Well, Brian did, and I went along mostly. There was this guy Billy who Brian knew from high school. He was this alcoholic with cancer and a colostomy bag, regularly on the verge of death, and he was out of his mind. He had wet brain from alcohol. His wife had divorced him when he was in rehab, sold the house, and gave him half the profits. Billy decided to buy a car, but he couldn't register it because of his DUIs. He asked Brian to register it, but he couldn't either because of DUIs—my wonderful boyfriend had hit an eighty-year-old woman and broke both her arms, but she told the judge to be lenient with Brian because he had a drug problem. That left me to register the car. When I did, I did it in my name. So it became my car. Billy used the car—a drunk guy driving a car that was registered in my name was not good, I knew, but then he went to jail. He'd given us his ATM card and PIN number so we could get him money when he was too sick to leave the house—he had $50,000 in the bank—and every day he was in jail, we took $400 from the ATM.

"When he got out, we conned him into entering a residential program. I used to visit him every day, and bring him shaving cream and magazines so that we could keep him there and use his ATM. I'd tell him, 'Don't leave. You have to get sober. We want you to be comfortable.' It wasn't very nice, but I was walking around with thousands of dollars in my pocket, and so was Brian.

"When Billy got out of his program and finally checked his bank account, he called the police on us. But what could they do? They told him, 'You gave them your card, and the car doesn't belong to you, it's in her name.' He calls up and starts yelling at me, 'You junkie bitch.'"

"That's one sad story," I said. She spoke as a detached observer, but insistent, too. She was very much alive while offering this account. It was as if she was interested in how mean and underhanded she'd been.

"It's ridiculous. Sometimes I think I should feel worse about it all. But what am I going do at this point? Who lives like that? You get into heroin and that kind of behavior's normal, unbelievably. When I understood that scamming people, robbing them, was just a given, I got fed up. I was at my worst on heroin. So I went back to Vicodin just before I came in here."

Every addict stops using for a reason; some aspect of life has become intolerable or torments them. But if Lucy had told me the Billy story on the first day she came, if she had explained that this was why she was "tired," I probably would have seen her very differently. Less sympathetically. Somehow Lucy had maintained an air of kindness and decency. But obviously she was not all sweet selflessness.

In the popular imagination, heroin is associated with crime. But in my experience, heroin isn't the issue, poverty is. And I've worked with plenty of addicts who were as poor as could be and made it a point to tell me that they never stole anything from anyone. Joe, my grateful handyman, had a moral code; if he had no money, he wouldn't eat for days until he found work, house painting or hauling trash. Marco thought criminals—though not opiate addicts—should be "locked up."

Whatever Lucy had gone through (and I hadn't heard even a small piece of it, I assumed) had been an ordeal, and the only prize, after ten years away from the upper middle class she had grown up in, was Brian.

"So where have you been staying since you got back from South Carolina? With Sean?"

"With him and some other friends."

"How's that been?"

"I have no apartment, no job, no money again, just like when I started with Brian. I have no jewelry. I sold it all to pay for the medication. I left everything when I escaped. I took a few records—yes, I actually own a few myself." Proud of being a little eccentric and out of the ordinary with her hobby, she smiled even in the midst of this horrendous story. "My Dylan and Beatles and Stones. I took a few clothes, one pair of shoes. I left photo albums my mother made for me—although she probably has copies of the pictures—and souvenirs from trips, and children's books I'd saved. I left my grandmother's Persian rugs with my criminal boyfriend. If my parents ever visit, and if I ever have my own apartment, I won't let them in. I want them to think I still have her carpets. It was my mother's mother's wedding gift. I wouldn't want to hear their scorn looking around at the few things I have and asking me why I don't have the beautiful carpets they gave me. I'll lie to my parents if they ever ask about it. I have no furniture, either. I left all that behind with him. I couldn't deal with going back for it once I was out. I actually feel worst of all about leaving my Burt Reynolds movie posters, which I'd had up on the walls of my room."

She stopped. As if she'd just heard all she'd been saying. She didn't want to be contemptible.

"I found an unopened package of cigarettes on the street today and I didn't take it. Imagine what it means that that's a good day to me," she smiled her bitter smile. "Three months ago if I found an *empty* pack, I'd have opened it and checked every centimeter of it. I found cocaine in a pack once when I was fifteen." She was proud of herself as a way to disguise her self-disgust.

Does behavior change by tiny inner shifts or seismic upheavals? With any patient under ninety years old, with any medical condition, I always feel there is a chance, there is hope, there is something positive I can offer. Even if the hope is getting to the next birthday, surviving until the next grandchild's graduation, having a month drug free. Even if the odds look miserably bad, there is hope. To tell patients otherwise is cruel.

"Sometimes I think it's easier to go back, give up, start again," Lucy said. "I'd have to deal with repercussions, though. At least when I'm not with Brian there's no screaming, no one stealing out of my pockets, no one around shooting dope.

"I feel isolated. I've felt isolated my whole life. These days, it's not in my head. The reality is, I am isolated. I never had a lot of healthy friends. I need to learn how to make healthy friends. I don't know any college-educated people. That's something of a challenge for me."

As I was writing out a prescription for buprenorphine and filling out the paperwork to schedule her next appointment for a month from now, Lucy was no doubt thinking about what she'd do when she left here and got back to wherever it was she was staying at this point. I am often aware that patients are waiting for me to approve or disapprove of what they've told me. But I didn't have the sense that Lucy was waiting. She was only pointing out her lack of life direction and the expected upcoming challenges. Maybe I liked her because unlike so many of my young, addicted patients, her prospects beyond her Vicodin-stunned days were not dishearteningly small. In the midst of her heart-wrenching confusion and dismay, she was thinking about college-educated people.

CHAPTER 6

Thursday, August 10

When I close my door after hours of interactions with patients, it seems unnaturally quiet for a moment until the men and women I've seen over the last few days appear in my mind. They are a line of expectant faces, nervous and awkward, offering good and bad reports. Their news—the death of a sister, the arrest of a son—is smaller than the news from the wars of the world, where the avalanche of the dead and missing crushes hope almost completely. My patients retain aspirations, and they bring their hopes to me; I listen to their news and do not despair. Perhaps I can help. I fear disappointing them.

If someone were to watch me from outside my window when I am alone, they would see me open a newspaper, look in my drawer for a piece of chocolate, or reach into my pocket for the paper with the phone number of a handyman who might help repair the broken shutters on the bay windows outside our dining room. Or I take out a shopping list to jot down a few things I've forgotten earlier—bread crumbs, limes. I write too quickly and my penmanship is poor to begin with, so even as I am adding items, I know that later, at the market, I will have trouble reading my scribbles below the rounder, fuller writing of my wife who has started this list. These chores are what I use at home to distract myself, what I use here as a defense, so that my mind is not suffused by grief and dismay. Unfortunately (and fortunately), I know what kills people, and I know all about the tests and difficult days before they die. A patient with liver failure from hepatitis C virus infection that I'd diagnosed died last week. I remember testing him years ago when I'd noticed bruising on his legs, a sign that his platelet count might be low. In testing him, I was going against his plan regarding his own health—if it's unnoticed, it will remain undiscovered (and magically go away)—but in fact he'd come into the office because of his fatigue, his inability to walk to work without stopping to catch his breath.

The nineteenth century is called the century of hygiene, and the twentieth is the century of medicine. The twenty-first century may be the century of behavioral change. Changing everyday, long-term behaviors—how we exercise, what we eat—is the key to adding years and quality to our lives. People find refuge in their habits, their likes and dislikes, just as I find refuge in my room, or in the monkish solitude of my research data or my shopping list. I understand how hard it is to change forty-plus years of smoking, thirty years of going to a bar on Friday and Saturday nights and forgetting to take medications on the following mornings, ten years of daily Vicodin use. There is no simple prescription. Every day I ask patients to interrupt the repetition of their habits. I ask them to sustain this interruption once they leave my room. I ask them to smoke less; to wear condoms. Men and women are greedy; they form desires early. They define their needs and protect them. Forcing the mind to do anything is nearly impossible. The mind is obstreperous. Even when shamed.

Although sometimes shame is enough.

When Julia first came to see me, she was ashamed that she could not get done what she used to—pricing new vendors, hiring new staff. She was ashamed that she didn't have the energy to do things at home. She was ashamed when her husband took their two daughters out for a day she had planned for the four of them together. "I couldn't wait to go back to lying down," she said. "I stayed in bed all Sunday until they came home. I didn't eat. I didn't take a shower all weekend."

She was mortified that her mother had discovered her problem. "My mother was always talking to other people as if me and my older sister were always sick. And my sister *was* sick; she had migraines. But even when we were well, things were awful. My mother became hysterical around my sister. She came off sounding like my sister was always about to die. My sister didn't have a life-threatening condition. She wasn't about to die. But my mother would cry as if she were. When I was eleven or twelve, I started to have terrible headaches, too, and I didn't tell my mother. I didn't want her hysterical around me, too.

"I had pain for two years, all day every day, before telling anyone. My grades slipped and my parents thought I was goofing off. After school, I would go to my room, close the door, lie down on my bed, and draw. There were fights at dinner. I wasn't hungry and I hid food in my napkin. They took me to a doctor and I didn't tell him about the pain, either.

"When I was thirteen, I finally told my mother about the pain and I started on medication for migraines and then I was much better. But after I was diagnosed, my mother wasn't interested in my schoolwork. If anything, she held me back. She never asked about school except to say, 'If you don't want to go to school today, you don't have to.' Even when I was well, she would say, 'You're in pain, right?' If I actually wasn't feeling well and I told her, she'd get so morbid. Sometimes, when you don't feel well, you just want someone to smile and say it's okay, right? She never smiled."

Julia was embarrassed by her years of deception as a child, and her deceit as an adult using opiates. But she was hesitant to blame her mother. She'd told me she was not someone who "blames her parents for her problems in life." She didn't believe there was anything she could do about her childhood now. But there were a lot of things she hadn't thought about since then.

"Whenever my mother would cry, she would have to take tranquilizers. She didn't hide them. My mother offered me pills for everything after she found out about my migraines. I took a school trip to Washington, D.C., on a bus when I was fourteen and she gave me one of her pills to take for the ride even though I didn't ask for it. She treated me for her fear. She was very protective. A doctor had once said that maybe some of my symptoms were related to nerves. Maybe my mother thought she was helping me. She offered me tranquilizers and I took them.

"Even now, when my mother thinks something's wrong, she'll say, 'You never tell me the truth, anyway. You keep things to yourself.' My friends would agree that I hide things well. My husband knew I was sick as a teenager, but doesn't know about my hiding it."

"I've made a mess of things haven't I?" she asked me, expecting disdain. "I didn't want to, but I did."

She didn't trust herself even after almost four months on buprenorphine. When I asked if she would use Vicodin if she had it in the house, she answered, "I don't know." Then she quietly said, "That's bad, isn't it?"

When I suggested that Julia start on a new medication, in addition to buprenorphine, that was known to have antianxiety and antidepressant effects, the first question she asked was, "Is it addictive, too?"

Julia had wide green eyes, a baby face, and a gentle expression. She looked as if she never stayed out past 11:00 P.M. Her voice was girlish and innocent of hardship. At her latest visit her hands were tense when she gripped the arms of her chair. Sunlight struck her hands and made her fingers glow red. She was on the verge of tears, and I had a rush of tender feeling.

Over the years, I've heard addicts say they had started Vicodin or OxyContin *because* they knew it was addictive. Everyone knew. Tom, my funeral director patient, was adamant on this point. He claimed he wouldn't have tried the Oxy or the Vic a second time if some part of him didn't want to become an addict. He didn't believe anyone who told a different story. The urge to become an addict, Tom believed, was either one of two things: a way to convince yourself you're immortal or a pleasurable way to kill yourself. He didn't accept that falling prey to addiction was a matter of low self-confidence or who your friends were. Tom wouldn't have believed Julia's story of a sinus infection leading to the unexpected effects of Vicodin.

Julia had been using Vicodin nonstop for more than a year when she came to see me. She wanted to stop because some aspects of her life had become intolerable. She didn't want to chase Vicodin or be chased by it any longer. She didn't want it to bother her anymore; she wanted to organize herself around something other than drugs. It was astonishing to me that she had lied to her parents and husband.

"I lied to doctors when I first started using a lot of pills. I had to pretend to be in pain. I wasn't very good at it. You'd laugh. I went to a few doctors, not many, and told them I had terrible back pain before I couldn't do it anymore. I was successful about three times. Then one doctor—you should have seen the face he gave me. He knew. I figured when I couldn't do *that* anymore, I'd just quit the drugs. But I couldn't quit without withdrawal. As I was running out of my last prescription, I started to wonder where I was going to get more. I had all these scenarios of how to get some. I'd hurt myself so that I'd have a valid complaint when I went to the emergency room. That was one of my plans. It was crazy. I'd think of people I knew who might have pain medicine in their houses. I didn't know anyone, but I'd go through whole lists of people in my head. Then I'd try to figure out how I would get into their houses and into their medicine cabinets. I couldn't stand that these thoughts would have such power over me.

"I had a neighbor whose husband's uncle worked with these guys who could sell you anything you wanted. It came up during lunch one day, how amazed she was that the uncle even knew such people. She didn't use drugs and her husband didn't, either. I asked her if she could get in touch with these guys so I could help my sister with her migraine pain. I used my sister as an excuse. She had her husband get in touch and that's how it went, from them to her husband to her to me, and I would send cash back through her.

"It went along for a while, then she stopped. She told me she wasn't going to do it anymore. She said my sister could overdose or get in trouble. She had questions for me about my sister that her husband had begun asking. I got nervous. He'd already cut down on what they let me purchase, although it was still a lot.

"When I first came to see you, my husband said I couldn't have contact with anyone who'd ever helped me get drugs. He thought

I'd been calling all sorts of people during the worst of it, and he went through my cell phone, but of course couldn't find any strange numbers, because it all happened right on our street.

"When I came into treatment and stopped asking my neighbor for pills, she had *more* questions, like, *What happened to your sister?* It was a good thing I stopped when I did. One of the three sources got arrested, one got fired from his job, and the third left the state. That's when I started having dreams about going to jail.

"I can't make the history go away. I wish I could erase the last two years. I get upset very easily—any TV show that mentions drugs bothers me. It reminds me of people I've lied to."

During her months with me, Julia had never returned to Vicodin, even as her depressive and anxiety symptoms increased. I admired anyone who could change her fortune around so sharply. When Julia was swallowing twenty pills a day, Vicodin devoured her world and left nothing in its place. She had had to overcome herself, rip herself free.

As I studied her round face at every visit, I was again and again astonished that she had lied to the people who loved her. My initial reaction was: Vicodin made her lie. The illegal purchase and use of Vicodin forced her to cover up. But I had learned over the years that I sometimes had the cause and effect backward. Opiates didn't *force* a person to be deceptive. Opiate addicts were often inveterate liars before they found opiates. Julia had perfected lying as an eleven-year-old. At every visit I wondered what else Julia wasn't telling me about her past. Had I learned the full extent of what she'd hidden?

This month's been good and bad," Lucy answered when she got into my office and I asked how she'd been. It had been five months since she'd begun my program, and now she came only once a month. One of the benefits of having buprenorphine pre-scribed in a primary care office is receiving a four-week supply, like a diabetic receives her insulin, or a hypertensive his blood pressure medication. Buprenorphine makes addiction just another medical condition.

Lucy lowered herself onto her familiar chair and gave me her profile. When she was not there, I could visualize the side of her face, the grainy skin, the start of the wrinkle line crossing her fore-head, but not her blue eyes, which so rarely met mine. Her nails were painted gold, and she was wearing white sneakers, Peds with yellow stripes, jeans, a white macramé belt that was too long and lay along her leg. Outside, the city was heating up. The white cross-walk lines under my window shimmered.

At her first visit, she'd moved like a lean, scurrying animal. More recently she'd come to each visit moving slowly, unsurely. I sensed she had nowhere else to go most days, that this was her only appointment. She had all day to sit with me. Other patients have an aggressive persistence; they want something and I offer benign advice in the grip of their ferocious waiting. Lucy only wanted to be treated fairly and she was never completely convinced she would be. She wanted to be forgiven and she wanted me to be the magnanimous one. Something had changed between us over the past few months: I was no longer irrelevant to her.

"I got a job," she announced. As always, she laid out the objects in a still life: her silver thermos, her purse of white uniden-tifiable material, her blue-gray scarf, her novel, this one by Toni Morrison.

"Fantastic. That's great," I said. Her good news was so rare, any scrap of it made me glad. "What kind?"

"At a pet store, Pets Plus. I needed the money because I got a new place to live, too. I moved into an apartment with two others girls."

"You found a place. That's great, too." I immediately wondered what she had told them. Her personal data was noteworthy, but I doubted she had revealed much. I wondered if Lucy's two roommates had drug histories themselves; maybe they were people she'd met while using.

"I have flowers in my new room and not much else. Every day one of my roommates brings home flowers for all of us from the florist she works for. And every evening it's quite a clean-up effort, but at least I have something to do. Twelve vases become twelve full garbage bags. I have no furniture except a bed and a little table. I can't get more unless I find a way to make fast money, and the only way to do that is to strip or sell drugs and I'm not willing to do either. Some people enjoy criminal activity, not me. Brian sold steroids and stolen car parts. I don't have the heart for dealing."

She laughed. It was good to hear her laugh. Had she been a stripper? The possibility had never occurred to me.

"It's not easy to get a job."

"You got an apartment *and* a job. That's a busy couple of weeks. Quite an accomplishment." Getting a job, or not losing the one he or she has, stabilizes an addict's life and a recovery. For addicts, a job surpasses any insight I could help them with in terms of making life possible again. A job—unspectacular but consistent—offers a setting they don't control and a responsibility to others and themselves they might not otherwise have, especially those who are single and childless, like Lucy.

"It's not easy to get a job when you've never really held a job," she said.

I knew she'd had only short-term jobs since college. I hadn't asked over the past few months what money she'd been living off since she'd left Brian—I figured maybe friends had been helping her, maybe her parents. (She wasn't charged for her visits with me; she had qualified, based on her latest income tax statement, for our hospital's program called Community Free Services.) She'd claimed more than once that she'd been looking for work, but I've wondered what patients like Lucy, who had no obvious responsibilities, do as soon as they leave my office.

"I mean I've had other jobs over the years. I've waitressed. I had a job as an aide at a day care center about five years ago. One day I went to work, passed out, fell on the floor. When I woke up—this was all before 8:00 A.M.—I sort of slunk away. I worked as a substitute teacher in a middle school. I had this one internship where I was actually fired for being sad. I remember the day. I had been asked to photocopy something and I did it incorrectly and folded it messily—it was supposed to be two-sided, but I hadn't listened and made it one-sided. This served as evidence that I didn't care about my work. I was using then, I'd called in sick a bunch of times, and my supervisor said, 'I've never seen such a sad girl.' It wasn't the first time someone had called me sad. The last job I had was at a dry cleaner's. It lasted a month, and that ended with an investigation by a detective. I *was* embezzling. But I didn't get arrested for it. If you're never caught red-handed, it's hard to press charges. All in all not much of a résumé, is it?

"Anyway, a few weeks ago I was looking at this clerking job over at the health department. It was the first time I've had to interview in a long time. Even as a kid, I dropped out before I was rejected. I was sensitive to rejection. I didn't compete if I didn't think I could win. I quit swimming, music, spelling bees. My parents expected me to be the best, but they didn't talk to me about why I wanted to quit.

"I didn't want to clerk once they started asking me questions. I felt like I was putting myself in a place that I didn't belong. I knew they wanted me to have some experience, so I gave them the name of a place I worked when I was twenty-two and told them it was more recent. I had to lie. I thought of coming up with something like, *I was raising kids and was out of the workforce*. I could have used that. I couldn't tell them the truth: that I might as well have never existed for the past ten years.

"So I left that interview and my first thought was maybe I should call Brian—even though I haven't talked to him since I moved out—and he can get me a few Vicodin from over on Broad Street, which is where he usually went shopping for my pills and his heroin. That was the sequence of thoughts—I'll never get a job, so I'll use again. But I also realized I haven't given it much time. I've dug myself a pretty deep hole."

It isn't unusual for addicts to be impatient. Even if they've used for ten years, many insist they can be done with buprenorphine in ten days. For those who push ahead with this time frame in mind, I am never sure if they are desperate to be helped or to be left alone.

"The pet store was just around the corner from where I live. I just walked in. I saw a HELP WANTED sign. I said I needed a job. Marie hired me. She's in charge. I lied to her, too. I said I'd just moved into the area; I made something up. She didn't ask much though. Why do you want to work here? she asked. I need a job, I said, I can work any hours you need, I told her. So you want to work here? Sure, I said. That was the whole interview. I started as a temp, but someone left the next day and now I'm full-time."

At the last few visits, Lucy arrived, sat, and started speaking. It was better than the alternative; many patients sat awkwardly, a bewildered quiet between us, as if fluid conversation was breaking some rule. Lucy rarely asked me a question. The pattern of our conversation was that if she slowed down or quieted, it was my signal to ask her another question that she answered readily. She was never in a rush for her prescription.

"Do you like the shop?"

"I'm happier when I work. I feel better. This may be pushing it a little, fifty-five hours a week, but I need the money."

"Fifty-five hours. No wonder you're tired. Where in the store are you during the day?"

"I work out front. Mostly phone and computer orders for now. Although as you know I have trouble with the phone."

"Yes. You mentioned that a while back."

"Marie wanted to know why I'm slow to answer the phone when there are calls. I even missed a few; people hung up before I picked up. It's not about the customers; I never answer *my* phone. I haven't answered it in weeks. I might as well shut it off. I just don't answer."

"Why don't you answer?"

She was quiet for a moment. There was the faintest change in her facial expression. An indentation appeared between her eyebrows. She was upset, unsure.

"There will be something awful at the other end. Some horrible unnamed thing." She stopped. The room was quiet enough to hear her breathing. Her eyes were down, troubled. The light caught only half of her face.

I remembered that at her last appointment her phone rang inside her bag but she didn't move to answer it. Most patients answered. I had a patient whose wife called during nearly every visit with me, reminding him to ask me something. "I'm with my doctor now. I'll call you back when I'm done," he would always tell her.

"It's not new," Lucy said. "This has been going on since I was eighteen. My parents used to have to call my college roommates to find out if I was alive, because I wouldn't pick up the phone. I just have this anxiety when it rings. I have no problem calling out, and caller ID works on my cell phone, but when I don't know the number, I don't pick up, which was a problem when I was looking for a job." She forced herself to smile at the absurd reaction to a ringing phone and the limitations it placed on her day-to-day life. "When someone called to interview me, or to set up a time for me to come in and I just didn't answer, I knew it was not going to help with my search for employment. I don't even like to check my messages. It's a problem. My parents call once or twice a week, and I pick up very rarely, and when I do, I always dread it."

"What's the dread exactly?"

There are many things patients tell me that I really don't understand because I've never experienced them. I have to wait for them to find the rights words to tell me the entire secret story.

"I don't know," Lucy said, looking away. I wondered if she did know.

I wanted to ask more, but sometimes I am curious about the wrong things, so I held back. She wasn't going to tell me about this part of her past yet.

"Louise, one of the girls with me out front, she knows I have a problem with the phone, and she tries to help. I stick with the Internet orders. I'm actually a very good worker. I'm responsible. I have a good memory."

"So there are some nice people working there?" It was important for her to know that I supported her sticking with a job.

"Actually, every one of them is mean to me. As the new person, I'm supposed to be there when they open and close the store, and I'm working weekends, and they still pick on me. I want to cry every day at work. It's awful. To treat anyone like they treat me is unbelievable. I do good work and they tell me I'm constantly doing everything the wrong way. Not the district manager. He likes me. But the other workers. 'You're too rough with the kittens,' Marie says. 'You talk too fast to customers,' Janice says. 'You're eating in the wrong place, move your food.' I let the women push me around there because I'm scared that I'm one bad word away from being fired, and then from being homeless, and going back to Brian and using again. I don't want to step out of line. It wouldn't take much for me to be in trouble, without savings, without any family living nearby."

"Does the stress bring on thoughts of Vicodin?" I asked. During our early visits, I progressed down a limited checklist of questions about her mood and her sleep and how these related to her craving or drug use. Having now seen her for months, having tested her urine and confirmed that she was drug free, I had shifted my interest to how the rest of her life might trigger relapse. To my thinking, relapse could be defeated in advance by regular, normalized talk of friends, family, and work.

"No," she answered quickly. I could see that she was thinking hard about what to say next. "Maybe for a split second. That's not true. Some days after work I start walking toward the south side where I know I can buy. See if my old friends are there. It's good that I don't have a car. I'm halfway there and I think: No, it's not about the drugs. It's just that I'm overwhelmed. I'm in a fight I can't win. I'm not sure what I want: To be happy or not to use drugs? To have a healthy, productive life? I get melodramatic. I start thinking I deserve to suffer for some reason, and then I start to believe it. Something will change if I make it another month, I think. Don't pick up, I say to myself. Then you'll have to tell him. Tell you."

I could imagine her taking the turn to the neighborhood only six blocks from the hospital. Past the Burger King and Empire Loan, past the Asian Food Market and the graveyard. Which street was the one where she would meet someone looking to sell

her a few dozen Vicodin? I could see her traveling toward her favorite dealers along a track she knew by heart from her time with
Brian, and before.

"Sometimes I think: it would be easy to get drugs now. It
wouldn't be easy actually. Brian had all the connections. I don't
even have anyone's phone number anymore. Actually, I might.
But then people like that don't keep the same number very long.

"So, yes. When I thought about drugs, did it last more than
a split second? It was actually pretty prolonged. It would be dishonest to say it was quick. But I'm a little saner now. I know
the consequences. Everything is difficult for me still. After all, I
wouldn't be getting abused by Marie eight hours a day if I didn't
have a drug problem."

Lucy wasn't speaking out of self-pity, but rather from exaspera-
tion. I liked her because she'd never let herself believe the standard drug addict fable: this young person could have been great
if she hadn't fallen.

"Work: that's a trigger, too. I used to always get high at work.
It was what I looked forward to about going to work. I still have
time to get high now. I could use during lunch. Get a little buzz
going during my private time. The bathroom at the shop is hard
for me. Every other job, I'd take my pills in the bathroom."

Buprenorphine controls opiate craving for most of my patients.
But for addicts who aren't taking buprenorphine, there are cues
(two people talking on a bus about detox, a particular song on
the radio, the smell of a hamburger) that elicit the same response
as actually taking an opiate (release of dopamine and other brain
chemicals). Craving is a form of memory. It is a reminder of how
important Vicodin has been to one's feeling of well-being.

"I'm not sure what's stopping me. I guess I don't want to crawl
back out of a hole. The way down would probably happen fast.

I don't have a safety net here anymore with my parents living in South Carolina. I have no family around. I used to be able to go to their house for days or a week if I needed a place to crash.

"When I imagine getting high on Vicodin, it's the first ten times I got high that I imagine, not the last seven thousand. The first few times I vomited and even that was sort of pleasant. I had no worries. I'd done every drug, but no other drug was as good as Vicodin. With a certain drug I felt creative but not productive. I'd think about things, but not do anything. On Vicodin, I had a better opinion of myself. It made me forget every problem I have or ever had. And it wasn't just the high. I felt good for two or three days after. Who wouldn't want to live like that?

"I still have all sorts of plots spinning in my head. I could go back to Vicodin, get a little high from that for a week or two. Plenty of people do that, don't they? Even after a few months on your medicine? Go on, come off. But for the piece of me that wants that, another part wants some achievements in life. I can't have both? Doesn't everyone want both? To be high all the time and to get ahead?"

She was right. Plenty of people go on and come off. To come off drugs, opiate users most often enter a three-, seven-, or thirty-day detox program that requires overnight admission to a facility, where they essentially take a break from life. Detox is one of the most common forms of alcohol or drug treatment in America, and it almost never produces long-term quitters. People talk about detoxing as a means of "getting it out of my system." But once liberated from a detox facility, nearly everyone goes right back on Vicodin or vodka. Insurance plans usually cover the days (offering payment for multiple detoxes a year) because they were time limited and relatively cheap. Detox is the insurer's way of saying: snap out of it, you can be done with Vicodin if you just take a week off. Although detox is a way of psychologically canceling the recent past by managing the immediate discomfort of withdrawal, it doesn't focus anyone on the future.

Lucy had been on buprenorphine for almost four months without a slip (at least I hadn't heard about one yet, and her urine results were all negative), and that was something to feel positive about. Even so, I couldn't predict if she would be drug free six months or six years from now. Her fate was determined by too many different factors: motivation, belief in her ability to maintain abstinence, whether she would hold her job, who her new roommates were, pride, luck.

"You've been sober for a hundred and ten days. How about that? That's pretty good." Despite her search for humor in most situations, it was difficult to keep Lucy positive for long. What she was trying to do—recover—must have seemed unrealistic, foolish, nearly impossible. I was proud of how she was doing.

Addicts often refer to their drug use as a "habit." But the word *habit* suggested something routine and easy, which drug dependence never is. Most habits became drudgery, but this particular drudgery is relieved by diminished consciousness. Numbness is adaptive.

"Okay, I haven't done drugs every day. Which is a turnaround from the 365 days of the year before I came here. But there's been nothing amazing. I don't deserve a reward. There's been no accomplishment, which is why I haven't celebrated. Maybe if I celebrated, I'd feel better."

Her smile was not quite earnest.

"So no celebrations, but are you doing anything for fun after work?" In other words, what was replacing the opiates?

"I went out last night, but it was pretty depressing."

I rarely feel my questions are exactly right, but sometimes they are terribly wrong. As Lucy started to speak, I felt that I had asked the wrong question. But what was the right question when life always felt like bad news to her? She had no feeling of well-being now that she had stopped Vicodin. Feeling good was a dream to her—she had to dream it up, and couldn't.

"I went to see some bands at the Mirabel Lounge with one of my roommates. There were all these happy people of roughly my age. They were having beers. I drank until I was twenty-one and by then I'd been banned from every bar in town for underage drinking or breaking bottles. I never noticed until last night that most people with beers are not really drinking. They take a sip or two and put the bottle down. They're not drinking alcoholically. Everything I did I had a problem with. I never drank in a normal way.

"Last night at the club, I felt left out of life. I felt jealousy and spite and anger and self-loathing. My roommate said, 'I feel so bad you're not drinking.' She didn't drink very much. She offered me a cigarette. I took a puff and it made me feel sick. I'm really losing my touch. She smokes, but not a lot. A pack lasts her a week. That's my dream, two a day that I could really enjoy. But I don't really understand how to do that.

"She's nice, fairly bright, interesting. She loved one of the bands; I didn't like it much, they were flakey. They reminded me of all the bands I saw in college, stupid antics that weren't very funny. Of course men came up to me, but who am I going to meet? What would I say: By the way I'm an addict? Where would I start really? The bass player from one of the bands came up to me. 'You from around here? Want a drink?' I don't even like people looking at me, let alone touching me. I found twenty dollars on the floor, that's the third time in six months I've found money. Must be a good sign."

"So the bar wasn't a trigger, either. No real drug temptation?"

"That I couldn't resist? Not really. I might actually have a life yet."

I nodded.

"There's still some corner in my head where I have the idea that using was better than it was, that I really enjoyed it, that it wasn't quite as bad when I didn't use every day, that it was kind of cool and exciting when Brian and I went to buy pills. That is the life where I belong. But enough bad things happened that I know how false that is."

Lucy couldn't forget the past, or treat it as a little mistake recently put right. Her strategy for coping with the breaking dam of drug-free life had been to keep busy at her new job. She didn't want to give herself too much time to think. She didn't want hours to reflect on what her boyfriend had offered, his concept of togetherness. Away from Vicodin, she hadn't really had time to consider what she liked, what she was good at. She had no idea. She had begun a job and found an apartment, but she had to reconstitute a complete existence. My heart went out to her— everything must have felt new and she had to do it alone.

"It is time for a change," a new addict had said to me the week before. But no one ever says that until something forces them to change. They say it to make themselves sound eager, ready, flexible, in control. And the change is not subtle for addicts. It is not a different taste in reading or a new appreciation of art. It is a matter of direction and orientation of life, the loss of a preoccupation, the taking on of new beliefs.

"Every day I worry I'll be fired even though I've done nothing wrong. I walk around the block for fifteen minutes before I can go into work I'm so worried.

"Actually, something pretty bad happened this week. This kid, this friend of Brian's, who from time to time has come into the store, came in on Friday at around two o'clock, drenched in sweat, pushing a stroller with his fifteen-month-old in it. He came into the store screaming my name, 'Lucy, Lucy, I have an emergency, I had an accident. I need a ride home.' My work colleagues knew him—he and ten other drug addicts I've known over the years and who are obviously homeless and fucked up have walked in from time to time. Every head turns when one comes in. You can smell them—stale smoke, dirty clothes. The whole atmosphere in the place changes even when they're not screaming. 'I'll give you a ride at 5:00 P.M.,' I tell Luther, just to shut him up and get him out of the store. 'I'll get Liam some candy and I'll come back,' he says.

"He shows up at 4:30. I ask Gina, one of the girls who works with me, if I can borrow her car. I don't even have an active license. I told my manager I needed to leave a little early, and now she's all sweet to me after our latest spat. She looked at the little baby and said, 'Make sure the child is safe.'

"As we leave the store, the front stroller wheels get caught in a crack in the sidewalk. Luther is pushing and screaming and rocking the stroller back and forth trying to release it. The kid is crying and Marie opens the door and says, 'I'm calling DCYF.' Luther turns around and screams back at her, 'You fucking bitch.' Marie looks at me again and says, 'Make sure that child's safe.'

"He has no car seat, but we get in Gina's car and strap the baby in the back. 'If that bitch calls DCYF, I'm gonna kill her,' Luther yells. 'I was molested when I was in DCYF. I'll kill anyone who calls them.' Luther's in the front with me, and as soon as he's in the car he starts tapping his pockets and saying, 'I can't find my $75 or my ATM card or my food stamp card.' He's screaming again.

And then the next minute he's nodding off, passing out. The kid is now screaming in the back. In a few minutes, Luther wakes up. 'Everything sucks. I'm a bad parent. I'm not a bad person.' Then he nods off again. When he wakes the next time, Liam is still crying and he says, 'I'm gonna give him to DCYF.'

"I already know that DCYF was involved when the boy's mother abandoned him, and they placed the kid with Luther. The third time he nods off and wakes up he doesn't even remember his son is in the backseat. The baby's screaming the whole ride.

"We get to his house and he jumps out without the kid, and goes upstairs, leaving all the doors open. What do I do? Leave? Call DCYF? I carry the kid upstairs and go into the apartment and put him down on the couch. It looks like every apartment I lived in for ten years, a complete mess. As soon as I put him down, Luther attacks me. He pushes me into a corner. He pulls my hair. He wrestles the phone out of my hand and throws it out the window. He's yelling, 'I see the way you're looking around. I have an excuse for being a junkie. I was molested. You're just a spoiled bitch with no excuse.' I tell him, 'You can hit me. It wouldn't be the first time I was hit in an apartment like this.'

"Someone must have heard the screaming and called the police. When Luther realized they were downstairs, he let me go. They came in—all the doors were open, they didn't even have to knock—and one picked up the kid. Luther starts telling them, 'Get this bitch out of here. She showed up at my work and followed me home.' They look at me and at him and they know he's lying. I don't stay around. I just leave.

"The whole thing freaks me out. I cried for a day. It was all a little too familiar to me. I felt his rage; the amount of rage in him was scary. It made me sad. I felt the whole human tragedy of this person's life and this kid's life. I felt bad for myself, because whatever I do, I still have folks like Luther showing up in my life. And he actually likes me and always has. For him to treat me like that . . . I shouldn't make excuses for him. But for some reason, I identify with him. I shouldn't, someone who mistreats women and children and himself.

"Anyway, the whole episode has made me and Marie friends now. She called me the next morning to ask about the child. I told her about the police. I have a good record working there. I don't call in and miss shifts with excuses."

I was out of breath listening.

"I knew Luther would be a problem the first time he came in. His voice was fucked up, and he was dripping sweat. And yet I said that very first time, 'Oh hi, how are you?' instead of throwing him out. I can't believe I let him into my work so many times. He was never more than an acquaintance, we were never close to begin with. But I've never said to anyone, 'I never want to see you again.' And I've had plenty of reasons. Luther's just another violent addict. Every addict I've known is violent."

"What would have happened if you'd said to him, 'Go away, you can't come back?'" I asked softly.

"I don't *know* why I don't feel I have the right to say that, even if I said it nicely. Do I like the attention?" She sounded miserable.

"Do you think you could say no to anyone from your old life?"

She paused to consider, then gave herself some credit. "Maybe I've been saying no more often than I think. I see this one kid on the street all the time when I'm walking home. I used to buy pills off him. 'My guy is still really good,' he whispers every time I pass by him. But I pass him every time. *That's* saying no. I can say no on the street, but it's trickier maneuvering relationships."

Her world was filled with drug offers, invitations, and intrusions.

"Like with Luther. Are there other people who are problems for you?"

I was expecting her to name Brian.

"Yes. Men. All men. I've always been with men who supplied me with drugs. Did I do what they wanted me to do? Yes. Was there any other purpose for my sexuality? No. That's what it was good for. Was I attracted to them? No. Would I have been re-volted by them if I were ever sober enough? Yes. Was I manipula-tive? Yes. I was far along the continuum of the sexual exploitation of myself. Was it poor behavior? Yes.

"I let myself be treated badly by men. It got more severe as I got older, but it was always there. The only men I can see myself with are addicted, not working, abusive. But I don't separate the men from the drugs. The attractive piece is the drug; the rest comes along." She laughed again. "I know that sounds ridiculous. I know I have to get past it.

"This is by far the longest I've been single since I was sixteen. Intuitively, it's the best thing I could have done. Now I have no drugs to come home to. I was oppressed, that's why I finally left Brian. I couldn't live like that anymore. No freedom. The only benefit was the drugs."

Many people see an association between sex and drugs. Some cocaine addicts use the same terms to talk about getting high and about having sex. Drugs are a release; getting high lets them lose themselves. Drugs, like sex, are literally self-annihilation, a form of controlled madness. Cocaine users particularly think that get-ting high offers a perception of acceleration, or of being drawn up into a speed and direction different from consciousness. It isn't dreamlike or hallucinatory; like sex, it is located in the body. It is mystical, spiritual, significant, but not dissociative. There is a surge of neurotransmitters, but which ones? The ones that come with terror and rapture? The ones that, like sex, involve the emotional parts of the brain—the amygdala, the nucleus accumbens, the brain stem as well as the cortex?

When taking drugs, my patients have told me, one feels life more strongly. But opiate addicts have *never* told me that their experience with sex was more powerful. None of my buprenorphine patients brag about their sexual adventures on heroin or OxyContin or Vicodin. Opiates actually make them feel unnaturally sluggish. Sex is an effort. They can't concentrate on anyone else, a prerequisite of good sex, when they are on drugs. Patients have told me that if their partner was high, too, it *seemed* like they were relating, but nothing was vivid. At best, sex was shadowy, colorless. Mostly, they weren't interested, or they didn't notice if they were interested. Vicodin shut down awareness in general. Yet sex remained dangerous, the only way to acquire HIV or hepatitis if you weren't injecting opiates. Not being interested in sex turns out to be protective for many of my patients.

"I have some good news for you," I told Lucy. She'd finally been to the lab a week before to have a blood test I'd asked her to have drawn at our second visit. She'd avoided it for more than four months because she was scared of hearing the result. "The blood work, the hepatitis C test, was negative. You don't have hepatitis C infection."

She started to cry. I'd never seen her cry. I was used to her unfocused gaze at the door, her tough-woman's nonchalance. I felt protective of her. I had the sense that whatever I knew about her life, I knew nothing about the worst parts. When she cried, it nearly brought tears to my eyes.

"My mother hated Brian. She knew he had hepatitis. I'd told her. Every time she calls she asks if I've seen him. She said she hopes he dies of hepatitis. It's hard to listen to your mother wishing for someone's death. I always figured he'd give it to me," she said slowly. "But I guess he didn't."

"He didn't." She had gotten the report of a negative HIV test just before she started with me, but hepatitis was what she most feared.

"That's another reason never to see him again. So I don't have to tell him that I got away without catching a disease from him. He'd probably wish I kept a reminder of him."

I felt an increasing sympathy and a sort of stunned admiration for her getting away from Brian and staying away. For lasting even this long on her own.

How long after she'd moved in with him had she realized that Brian was mean, careless, harsh? Constantly worried about the risk of withdrawal, her default position had been to continue with him for nearly two years, to accept him as her source for opiates. When she was desperate, he didn't alarm her; for a decade she had not even tried to save herself. She didn't feel good about herself, why would she feel good about the man she lived with? I wondered if she could even discern kindness.

"The best part of being clean is staying away from men. I saw some younger girls coming out of a meeting the other night who haven't figured that out yet, and I felt bad for them."

"Have you heard from Brian?" I asked.

"He's been calling, but I don't answer. He calls me about four hundred times a day, first from the hospital and now from my former home."

"Have you been back to the apartment since you left?"

"No. But he keeps calling."

She stopped speaking, pursed her lips, and blew. She made no eye contact. "I erase all the messages on my cell phone. When I was younger I thought my whole family was going to die and that at any moment I would get a phone call about it. They weren't dead yet, and I would have to pick the order: who would die first. Not only would I not pick up the phone, I was afraid to leave the house. I had rituals to protect people. If I counted all the letters in the last sentence I'd spoken before the phone finished ringing and it was a multiple of three, my mother wouldn't die. I still count now if I'm nervous."

I knew Lucy had not been a conventional teenager. She had been more than unreachable and moody; she had been in trouble. It sounded as if her troubles had started even before adolescence. My silent thoughts turned to the question anyone would have had: What had her parents failed to provide?

"Between when I was five and eight years old, both my father's parents died, and an uncle and cousin. Every time my father picked up the phone, it seemed to me, someone died. I had nightmares: in one, I was dead and looking at my grave; I'd been electrocuted. I had insomnia. My parents knew I couldn't sleep, couldn't fall asleep, but they didn't know the severity; they made light of it. My father would say to my mother: *she's so smart she must be awake thinking in bed.* I was miserable at a time when most kids are miserable, but I took it further. My parents remember me as happy. I must have hid it well, or they tried not to notice.

"Now I don't answer the phone because I'm afraid people are hunting me down."

My neck prickled, my skin seized. I could feel sweat on my back. Lucy wouldn't pick up the phone; were her reasons irrational or rational? Was Brian stalking her?

"Who?"

"I don't know."

She shut her eyes, a rare sign of stress. She didn't want to speak about Brian or sadness anymore. Her world, the world of men, had not been good to her. I wondered whether she expected me to be. I wondered if, underneath the chatter and bravado, she was terrified of me. I didn't believe she was, but she could be difficult to read. She had no one else to talk to about her life.

"My mother wanted to give me a good life. But she couldn't.

She had some success with my sister. Did I tell you she's getting married?"

"I don't think you did. When will that be?"

"About three months from now, the first week of November, in South Carolina, near my parents' place."

"She's younger than you are, right?"

"Four years younger. My father thinks she's spoiled, but my mother made my father agree to have the wedding in South Carolina. That's what she told me right before she told me she wants me to go back to school. I've had a job for a month and she wants more. She doesn't know I don't have money to go to school even if I wanted to."

Even after months, I couldn't tell if Lucy had a safety net, whether her parents were ready to help if asked. Had they written off the commotion of her life or hoped the entire time that she'd come back to face the world of living, working people?

Many addicts completely antagonize their families—stealing from them, lying to them, compromising them in ten different ways. With the loss of family comes a certain lack of accountability, I've found, because parents, siblings, and spouses are not only a source of support, but are also the embodiment of the idea that one is part of something greater than oneself.

"But you're paying for an apartment. Tell me about it."

"It's this great place with a double parlor and big rooms. We each have a bedroom. We share the kitchen. The two other girls have been there six months. They didn't know each other before they moved in. They seem to like me. I signed my own lease though. I don't really trust other people. I know what I've done with other people's rent money over the years. I'm more comfortable paying myself rather than pooling our money. My nightmare is to give rent to a roommate for three months then find myself evicted when the landlord hasn't been paid."

Addiction is brain chemistry and life circumstance and a system of thought and a way of being. People change their behavior the way a train moves along a track. Sometimes one crawls along before getting up to speed. Sometimes work is being done to the track and one stops completely or even reverses. Sometimes one abandons forward movement after a bad, bumpy ride—feeling discouraged and despairing—and gets off. Sometimes one gets through the tunnel.

When she saw me reach into my pocket for the prescription pad, signaling I had to see the next patient, she slowly gathered her things—book and thermos and purse—but kept talking.

"My landlord is hitting on me. He's married. He's twenty-five years older than me. He's been making it clear that if I don't want to pay him, I don't have to if I sleep with him, and amazingly, I've been considering it. It would make my whole life easier. Free rent. In my mind, it would be like I'd finally be getting something for being exploited my whole life. He's a shady guy. I feel unsafe. I keep waking up at night hearing people coming in through doors. It is possible; he has a key. I don't think he'd do it, though. In all my years using drugs, the option of trading sex for housing never came up.

"I won't do it, of course. 'The whole thing devalues me,' I told him. 'It feels like prostitution.' 'Well, you could still pay me the rent then,' he said. 'That's not going to happen, either,' I told him.

"Why me? Why did he ask me?" Lucy asked beseechingly. "My sister's getting married and this is who I'm left with."

"Do you think he's asked your roommates?"

"The very first time I met him, he complimented me. He said something like, 'It doesn't have to be like this.' So why me? Does he know something? Do I exude something?" She spoke haltingly, angrily. "He owns like twenty buildings. There's no way he hasn't made the same offer to others, and maybe some of them accepted. But why did he pick *me* out? Do I walk around with a sign that says, Abuse me?

"One reason not to accept is that if I had the extra $300, I'm sure I'd treat myself to drugs. That's the main reason not to agree to his kind offer."

That's the main reason not to accept? I wanted to scream to wake her up. She was two selves—the one who was now working and looking forward, and the other who was convinced she was worthless and hated herself for it. No wonder she couldn't look at me. It was torture to remain in the room with someone who knew about the way she lived. I could imagine her landlord's lusty, grinning eyes. Three hundred dollars, her share of the rent, must have seemed an enormous sum to Lucy.

"He must think I'm vulnerable enough to do it," Lucy said, "and that he'd get away with it because he must also think I wouldn't tell his wife. She deserves a phone call and a warning if he does shit like this. He rents mostly to women, it turns out. There are six apartments in my building and only one of them has any men. But what I want to know is: What's he reading on me? That I'd let him get away with it? That I'd let him victimize me and I'd shut up? I *know* I'd buy drugs because I'd have to be high to sleep with him. What a disgusting thought."

I'd asked her at our first visit, "Were you ever abused, physically or sexually?" She'd been adamant in her denial. But I knew her better now; perhaps she would be willing to admit to that awful history.

"You know the sad part? I actually did a quick assessment: Is he violent? Obviously there's some coercion in finding younger women to go after, there's some violence in that. But I figured he wasn't violent; he was too wrapped up in his social standing to risk that, and he was worried about his wife hearing about it.

He's not a violent rapist, just a coercive bastard. But really, is there much of a difference?

"I actually thought about going through with it with him, but I held off. Maybe if there were more money involved." She laughed bitterly again, but I could tell she was almost serious. "I can't do behaviors like that. I know. I might not be happy or completely well, but my life is a tiny bit better, and if I want to live, I can't do stuff like that. Why do people pick on me? In the drug situation I can see why—just being a woman by definition makes me vulnerable. But why would he?"

"Because he's a bastard," I said. I could feel her look over at me, but I'd lowered my eyes.

"I really didn't want to come today. I thought of using before I came in, even though I knew I wouldn't get high because of the buprenorphine I took this morning. I have an urge to punish myself. You're going to find out I'm a horrible person."

"I'm glad you came, even though it's been a bad and good month. And I'm glad you didn't use." With every patient I wondered: Do I actually know the things I think I know about you? Your life outside this room is filled with people I've never met and will never meet. After months with Lucy, I felt for the first time that I'd gotten a full dose of her life outside.

Later, as I was driving home, I thought for a long time about why Lucy avoided my eyes. We had had almost no eye contact during our visits. Did she not want to see my reaction to her words? My understanding of this strange lack of connection had changed over time. I had wondered during her first visit if she had even been listening to me. I'd thought that her staring at the back of my door, rather than even looking over at me, was meant to be off-putting and distancing. A refusal to meet my eyes said, Stay Away. A glance would expose her.

When I saw her during withdrawal, I presumed that she was affecting casualness. Not looking at me was a sign of inwardness. She closed her eyes as a last refuge, a final defense when the pain was hideous. She closed her eyes to think about something else.

But more recently I had begun to wonder if she even realized that she was picking a point on the wall to look at rather than look at me. Was she even doing it on purpose? She barely looked at me when *I* was talking. But that could have been because my gaze reminded her of how badly she felt about herself. Or perhaps she thought that as a doctor I would see right through her. The exchange between doctor and patient is always prurient because it is the passing of secrets from one stranger to another. Did Lucy hide her eyes as a way to tell me she had more things to conceal? I had not known her for very long, but I was also no longer a stranger to her. My attention and concern were real.

Maybe to meet a stranger's eye for too long was seen as a form of defiance by jealous boyfriends, and she didn't want to be accused of staring because it would lead to being hit. Was meeting the eyes of a man in a small, closed room a form of surrender? Would a female doctor have been a more comfortable choice for her? Or was speaking with any doctor too awkward, too revealing, too upsetting and embarrassing, too intimidating and intrusive?

Lucy had ten events a day that could trigger hopelessness in anyone: mean-spirited coworkers, unwanted and violent drug users wandering into her store and making demands, a vile landlord. A convoy of bad news and tough choices headed straight at her all the time. No wonder she looked weary. It was an impossible struggle, and yet probably better than any week when she was taking Vicodin and living with a heroin addict. Now that she wasn't using, she couldn't get away from her past.

CHAPTER 7

Wednesday, November 22

It was a snowy, cheerless day. I wanted to go home, get in bed with a book. I looked out the window and shivered. I could see five floors down outside the emergency department, dry, capped heads through translucent umbrellas. Heavy snow hit and ran down. Boots left prints. I wanted to get out of town.

Whenever I look at a day's schedule, I try to remind myself that each interaction—and with new patients who are shopping for a doctor there might be only one encounter—should be positive, stabilizing. My only responsibility toward patients is to try to leave them better off than I find them.

When I went down the hall and poked my head into the waiting area to look for Lucy, I felt I'd done my job with her so far. The TV was on loudly in the corner. Every eye was on it—nothing could make them look away from the nonstop tragedies and scandals of local news.

Lucy wasn't interested in other people's lives, including mine. She was learning to be more interested in her own life. She was getting better. On Vicodin she hadn't expended much effort doing anything, including trying to save herself. She'd had no steady work, no friends, no plan, no vision of life. Brian and other men who came before him had insulated her from making decisions. She took what came her way. Almost nothing alarmed her. An outside observer would credit her with improvement during her months with me. She felt better, but life, available again, seemed too large, almost out of reach. How did she know what she wanted?

I had been seeing Lucy for more than half a year. Although she was not in one of my research studies, most clinical protocols testing new treatments for drug users end after six months. Researchers usually wrap up their clinical trials (I am no exception) at this point. Because the time frame of studies is limited, relatively little published data exist about how addicts do over longer periods, and so we have come to equate treatment success or failure at six months as a final state, the primary data point, beyond which we can only guess. The six-month horizon is not only in keeping with financial realities of research grants, but also with even skeptical researchers' desires to believe that therapies work fast. If a treatment hasn't worked after six months, who has time to wait? And if it has worked, it will likely continue to work, following this line of thinking. But the permanence of any addiction outcome is illusory. If Lucy had been in one of my studies, I appreciated, I wouldn't be seeing her anymore; her study would be over. But she wasn't, and I was glad she was here so that I could see what would happen with her in the months to come.

She walked quickly to my office a few steps ahead of me. Inside, she crossed to her chair and laid her book and purse on the floor. Seated, she lifted herself and tucked her legs under her. Her pose was lax, docile.

"How was the wedding?" I asked.

"It was horrific."

"Horrific?"

"I hadn't seen any of my family, my cousins, my uncles, since my grandmother died three years ago." She adjusted herself, collapsed into herself, chin on chest, knees up so I could see skin above her squeezing sock line.

"Okay."

"I was never close to anyone in my family. I wasn't looking forward to seeing anyone. But I was ready for all the questions. When are you getting married, when are you going back to school? I'm a good talker. I can keep the conversation going and superficial. But no one at the wedding would really talk to me. There was silence all around me. Everyone avoided asking me anything. No one asked me a direct question."

"What do your relatives know about your life these days?"

"I didn't know who knew what. But I felt I had nothing to say. Could I really walk in and say, 'Hi everyone, I'm almost six months clean?'"

"That would have been a tough party opener. So let's move on to something more important," I said. "What did you wear?"

She liked the question, raised her chin, staring at the back of the door. "My sister said I looked good. Which I did. A teal dress. Gold heels. I paid for it, although my mother contributed. Now, at least, I own a dress."

Lucy's visits almost always started happily. I could see the child in her face, the buried life rising to the surface, the fear and pride. There was a lightness in her mouth and eyes, a sweetness, but the pattern of these visits was that the longer she spoke, the more she revealed and the sadder she became.

"That's excellent. A dress will come in handy at the next big occasion."

"But still I didn't think I was dressed appropriately."

"It sounds like you were."

"At a lot of weddings, the hosts buy outfits for everyone in the wedding party, right? I wasn't even *in* the wedding party. You think my sister or her husband would put me in the ceremony? When she was planning the wedding, she probably heard I was in a program, and I'm sure she didn't ask what kind and I doubt my mother even remembered. No, my mother just wanted to make sure I looked okay, so she sent me some money for a dress. I didn't want her to pay at all. I've already used her money for a college education, to avoid eviction when I was with Brian, and for Vicodin when I was in a pinch. But I couldn't afford to buy a dress for myself."

"So you let her pitch in."

"I'd already spent all the money I had on the airplane ticket."

"It must have cost a lot to fly down."

"It's not only that. I had to miss a week of work. I can't afford to miss a week of work. As of last week I had $231 in the bank. That's all I had to my name."

"Every expense must feel enormous."

"I didn't get a haircut. My mother offered to pay for that, too, but I wouldn't let her. Anyway, I'm weird about haircuts, I don't like people touching my head."

"It's always sounded to me as if your mother never minded helping financially."

"Having her money over the past few months has been the only reason I'm not hopeless. But I'm guilty about having accepted money in the past for things she didn't know I was using it for."

I thought of another patient of mine who started each visit saying, "Same old problems, family and money. Too much of one, not enough of the other."

I found myself addressing Lucy as if she were a churlish fifteen-year-old who was balking at a necessary fact of the world. I often hear from colleagues that they treat addicts like adolescents. Common wisdom suggests that addicts, no matter how old they are, have the maturity of teenagers. Somehow they all get stuck at the age of vanity and irresponsibility and never progress. Like any adolescent, addicts have no idea of the risks they are taking, and if they do, they are proud of their bad behavior, proud of not being afraid. Addicts are willful and deeply resentful of the slightest interference or objection, so of course they can't hold jobs. They become daredevils in certain ways, secretive in others.

I remembered girls like Lucy Fields from my large urban high school. They weren't troublemakers or class clowns, but they had somehow removed themselves; they were in retreat, not engaged, dressed in carpenters' pants, almost trying to look penniless. They made their discomfort seem natural; if I'd looked closely, I might have sensed their unease. We called them "wasted" while they looked with amused bafflement at boys like me who must have seemed serious and aloof. Twenty years later the word *wasted* seemed right; Lucy had wasted her gifts, her intelligence. Like any teenager, when she started drinking vodka and getting high on cough syrup, she had no idea how it would mark her. She'd found drugs irresistible, but wasn't it a sign of youth to find anything irresistible? The string of circumstances and choices that triggered and nourished her becoming a full-blown addict kept her, in some ways, in adolescence. Addiction, like adolescence, represents forces that tug against rationality.

Not every addict acts like a teenager. But the ones who arrive late and look at me as if I am an idiot when I tell them to reschedule make me want to say, as I did to my own teenage children, who have given me the same look, "It's your fault. Don't come crying to me."

I remembered thinking during her first visit that Lucy's obscured view of the future was very adolescent. Drugs were in her way and she couldn't see through them. Today again she had an adolescent's aspect, facing the door and not me, barely raising her chin when she spoke.

"How was your sister?" I asked.

"She's excluded me from family life for years. I guessed this would be more of the same, even though she had to invite me. Her husband talked to me more than she did. My sister and I did talk when I first got there. She asked me about my job. I guess I'm not quite the disappointment I was, now that I have a job. It wasn't much of a conversation—I'm not that interested in talking about work—but I'm not sure what I wanted to say. I don't know if we have enough in common to have a real conversation. She told me about her law school applications and her personal statement, which I was just thrilled to hear," Lucy said sarcastically. "Her husband went to business school so I guess she's trying to compete. The day before the wedding my sister ran a 10K road race down there. I don't believe the human body is meant to do things like that, but anyway, she always does her competitions for some charity. I donated five dollars to her lymphoma research cause. I was very proud of giving her money that I'd earned. My five dollars was like someone else's five thousand dollars."

Lucy had always been different and must have suspected there was something wrong with her from an early age. Her sister was the representation of all that was normal; she'd told me as much.

"The morning of the wedding my sister yelled at my parents for two hours for not coming to her race, and how wonderful her husband's family is because they knew to come, and how crazy ours is. My parents said they didn't know how important the race was to her.

"Her charity is lymphoma research because of my mother. My sister wrote this moving story on her website about the insidious disease of cancer. It was a really long piece; she must fancy herself a writer. From the story, you'd think she grew up in a family of three. There was no mention of a sister. No mention of my name. She must not realize that she completely left me out. She was obviously very proud of what she wrote. She actually showed me the site and asked me to tell her what I thought of it. I didn't say anything. My father noticed that I was left out, too. Could it really *not* have been conscious on my sister's part? 'My mother's courageous battle against cancer, her ability to hang on through side effects.' I couldn't believe it. It certainly wasn't like that picture she drew in kindergarten: mom, dad, my sister, and me. I thought of writing an anonymous reply to her site: Don't you have a sister? Did I really deserve to be completely omitted from the family history?"

The bright winter light gave Lucy a hard radiance.

"Even if she'd written, *I have a troubled sister.* Come on. The omission is pretty striking. Also, her family has been affected by more than one illness. She probably doesn't think of it that way. Maybe she only counts nondrug illnesses like cancer. She probably thinks I chose, or choose, to inflict harm on the family, even if harm was done to me, too. She has pretty conservative political and social views. I can hear in her voice that she probably thinks I'm just a loser or consciously chose to hurt others. Which is not true. I don't know what I can do at this point to change that. She knows I'm doing better. But did she know how bad it was? I've had very little to do with her during the last decade. I went to her college graduation, but only by accident; I happened to be home that weekend, trying to borrow money from my parents. I used to think of plausible stories about my life. I didn't like her looking down at me so I made everything up. Where I was working, who I was living with? There was usually a grain of truth in what I said. For a while, I would try to keep up on my lies to be consistent, but I gave up on that. I don't know what she knows about what I've been doing during the past ten years. Does she think I was sick or just ignoring her?

"I didn't want to get into that discussion with her at the wedding." She went slack and sat heavily, a desperate-seeming posture.

"How was the ceremony?"

"You want the gruesome details? Here's how it was for me: I see my sister and I'm resentful and self-pitying."

"Resentful of what?" I could imagine but wanted to hear.

"Let's start with the fact that my sister and her businessman husband paid for the whole thing for a hundred people."

"Your parents probably helped them, too."

"I don't think so. Last month, I was keeping money under my mattress and didn't even have enough to open a checking account. I pay my rent in cash. How humiliating is that? A person doesn't pay rent with cash or a money order. I wasn't raised that way."

Lucy had lived in circumstances far beneath her for years, daughter of two professionals that she was.

I tried to steer her away from self-pity. "Do you like the man she's marrying?"

"Do I like her husband? Doug? He organized the speeches and he could have involved me, his wife's only sister. But he didn't. So no, I don't like him much. You know what he says to me after the wedding? 'Come visit us. I'll pay.' A little rude and presumptuous, don't you think?"

Not presumptuous, generous, I thought. Obviously Doug knew the score. He knew that his new sister-in-law was short on cash. Lucy was a stranger to herself, but she was revving up, getting angrier and angrier. Her small hands flashed in quick movements.

"Had you met him before?"

"Just once. When I was using. At a family party about three years ago. That was an awful day. I'd just had a fight with my boyfriend. Did I ever tell you about him, the guy who broke a mirror over my head? He was the guy who would sit and watch me at work at the Laundromat for seven hours, then go out and cop for us, and then come back and accuse me of cheating on him during the fifteen minutes he was gone. That evening, before the party, he accused me again of being with another man and locked me out of our apartment. I went to the party alone and as punishment, the next day he took my money, my bank card, and my pills. He left me drug sick. At the party, I was quiet and stayed for only ten minutes. My sister drove me home and my mother told me she was in tears when she got back."

"Did she ask you what was up with you at any time during your three days in South Carolina?"

"She's never asked. She's never confronted me." All her family's energy went into *not* noticing Lucy.

"And she wasn't very nice to you at the wedding party either, you said."

"My sister didn't say anything to me that she wouldn't have said to anyone else who was there. She didn't say anything personal. She was just one of a group of happy, normal, privileged people.

"My parents were nicer to me than my sister was. My sister has a condescending streak. My mother says it's not just directed at me; she doesn't return her phone calls, either, and when she does, my mother told me, she always says, 'I'm very busy. We have to keep this short.'"

Lucy had done things beyond apology, failed friends in large and small ways and I presumed failed her sister, too, which was not easy to undo. I could imagine Lucy suffering through the wedding. The day must have provoked in her a confusion of feelings—helplessness, rage, sadness, doom.

I could have asked her more about her sister and the day she cried, or I could have asked more about the new husband, but I asked something about the food they served.

"It was actually good. They had two entrees. I had the vegetarian lasagna. My sister is a vegetarian. I'm not short, but it felt like the cousins and aunts at my table were talking over my head." She laughed mildly, sadly. "Eleven people at my table and not one asked a thing. They probably heard about me and didn't know what was safe to ask. Not even where I worked or lived. I wouldn't have told them, anyway. I'm not sure they could have taken it at the happy occasion. I snuck out for a cigarette about five times."

What else did she sneak out to do, I wondered?

"Tell me why you couldn't announce to the table, 'Hi, I'm six months clean?'" I was challenging her. I rarely played devil's advocate.

"I guess I could have. Some addicts I know have done that at family occasions. They think: this is the way I am, take me or leave me. I could have done that at the wedding with my aunts and uncles and cousins. But instead I thought: no one really knows about me. How much do they need to know? I don't have relationships with any of them. What do I care what they think? I don't get credit for being like everyone else and why should I?"

I understood well enough what she was trying to say. She was ashamed of using Vicodin and she was ashamed of using buprenorphine. With both, she worried about being found out. She wasn't a very good actor. Although she felt out of control, she disliked drama and abhorred the overly emotional. It struck me that I would have done exactly as she had done if I were in her position at the wedding: I would have said nothing to the other guests. But in my office now, she also went silent, her shoulder twitching. It was not unusual anymore that she would break off in the midst of saying something, go still, staring blank-eyed into the nothing of the door, as if she could hear some distant alarm I couldn't. She had a shallow way of breathing, never even a deep sigh. After a few minutes, the silence began to swell, creating a pressure against both of us.

"My father was in a bad mood. But he always is. My mother seemed miserable, and she's usually the upbeat one. She turned to me during the wedding and said, 'I won't live to be old and I want to see you have a career and your sister to have children.' She's in perfect health, but all weekend she told me she's dying. My mother was sick years ago, her prognosis wasn't good, but she's fine now. It's true that her support group from when she had lymphoma are all dead except one, a good friend of hers ever since, who came to the wedding even though she's *really* sick, rediagnosed three years ago and still getting chemo, but with cancer all over her body. Maybe that's it. Maybe that's where the line about dying came from. Did she say this to make sure I would be nice to her? I didn't know whether to laugh or cry. Maybe she sort of believes she is dying. I didn't know what to do.

"I know how to do drugs, that's what I know."

It was a thought she didn't need to finish. Even after six months with an addict it was ludicrous ever to feel triumphant.

"You used?" Wasn't that what she was trying to tell me?

I waited for the little grimace that signaled agreement. She was looking at the floor when it appeared.

"I did."

One part of her wanted to continue to talk in her outspoken way, pretending there was nothing wrong, but another part had to withdraw, and she braced herself, reorganized herself on her chair. It is commonly believed that addiction hollows the user, leaving him or her shamed, lethargic, dull; it creates a surrounding indifference. But Lucy didn't seem indifferent at all.

"What did you use?"

"Vicodin."

I can never see what is coming, although giving advice every day to strangers makes me start to believe I can. My disappointment, which was lined with irritation, shocked me. It was a piece of metal caught in my throat. I should have known trouble was coming; I know so little of their lives outside my office. Even while hearing the details of the wedding weekend, I wasn't sure that I could ever understand what led up to the moments before Lucy used. These moments are the centerpieces of the stories addicts tell each other at NA meetings, cautionary tales, senseless, wrapped in bewilderment.

"When did you use?" There was an edge to my voice; it would have been awkward pretending nothing was wrong.

"The day of the wedding. I skipped my buprenorphine that morning."

The way she said it made clear she regretted it all now, but also that the wedding day Vicodin had been premeditated. Her slip took some planning; she'd had to find some Vicodin. She had not used buprenorphine because it would have blocked the Vicodin effect, the day's high. I understood the pharmacology of buprenorphine, its chemical properties, its formulation, its long half-life, but there was no fact about it that helped me understand why she had used Vicodin again, took the risk of spiraling back into her hole. I thought about the joke Lucy once told me about how when a normie's car breaks down he calls a towing service, but when an addict's car breaks down, she calls her dealer. To stay sober, each day the addict has to say to herself, "No matter how awful I feel, it's not as bad as. . . ." That had worked every day for six months for Lucy. But in South Carolina, she wanted to check out for a few hours. Sometime before, during, or after the ceremony she decided to disappear, to go invisible, to vanish from her life, not by leaving Hilton Head, but by staying where she was in a different way. She didn't want to participate in other people's pleasure any longer. She wanted her own. A delicious break was all she needed. Melting into a chair, letting the South Carolina warmth join the Vicodin warmth seeping into her bones. Erasing herself.

"Did you make it through the wedding?"

I could see she was embarrassed—she didn't know what to say, how much, how to behave. "Almost. It was eight at night and everyone was dancing and I was looking at two more days with my parents and I needed something to break the fast-approaching monotony."

She didn't wait for me to ask why? She knew I would. She had a measure of me, no doubt, after all these months. There were a finite number of plausible excuses for her slip, and she chose boredom. This was one version, an insufficient one. But relapse is never about boredom and monotony; it is about feeling badly, or badly about oneself. Trapped with her parents, I'm sure Lucy was grateful for any excuse to get away, if only for a few hours. She didn't need to look far for ten other reasons, besides a few more days with her parents.

"So you used at the wedding."

"I stepped away from the festivities for an hour or so. I'd seen too much of my family."

Some people, nonaddicts, at their sister's wedding, stricken by melancholy or anxiety, would have taken a long walk, or offered to drive older relatives back to their hotel, or had a drink. Lucy wanted to close her eyes and grieve, and the way she knew to do this was to take Vicodin. She wanted to check out for a while, not feel overwhelmed, lonely, angry. In South Carolina, she didn't want to feel any feelings. She needed to shut down. She wanted relief from reality.

As Lucy spoke, I found myself more and more disappointed with her and I tried to beat it back by telling myself *Yes, yes, yes, of course, this is what addicts did.* Sobriety is hard to implement. Simple, absolute sobriety, forevermore, is nearly impossible. But is it? Was forcing myself toward calm acceptance of this impossibility a nod toward helplessness? Was I as hopeless as Lucy Fields had been that morning in South Carolina? Had I presumed there would come a day like today when we would deal with her relapse, almost as if it were inevitable, as if it were assigned to her?

I was disappointed. I blamed her for not struggling enough, for not recognizing the perils. For Lucy, every morning brought the daily decision: use today or don't. Each day, holding off relapse had to be an improvisation. Sometimes she did it for herself, sometimes she did it to reconnect with her parents, and sometimes, I liked to believe, she did it to please or heed me. It worked for a while, then the need piled up. I wondered if she brought a few Vics with her, or if she'd gotten them while she was in South Carolina, maybe from a distant cousin she met at the wedding.

Eleven million epidemiologically demonstrable (it's impossible to prove the accuracy of such figures) Vicodin users make addiction a peculiarly common modern American condition. Of course someone in the wedding party had a few pain pills on him or her. This may not be a comforting thought for public health experts, police officers, or even drivers on the road, but as a doctor it doesn't surprise me.

"Did you go to a meeting again?" I was wondering how she had stopped herself, prevented the first snowflake from becoming an avalanche.

I thought about the trip she took to South Carolina just weeks after starting with me, when visiting her parents was a way to get away from Brian. She had been to an NA meeting that time in Hilton Head, five months ago, and had complained about it. Mutual help group ideology had it that in recovery the addict is powerless before a drug's temptation. To have a chance, one needs to submit, surrender one's will to a higher power. Although NA does not mean this submission as a way to absolve oneself from taking responsibility, I worry that for some of my patients it encourages invalidism. Helplessness appeals to some people. It automatically confers sympathy. Yet I saw these months of Lucy's sobriety as an act of will, not the surrendering of will. I wanted her to be willful. I didn't want her to feel acted upon, a victim of her family. Doctors do best when their patients are motivated, participatory, disciplined.

"I told you, I can't stand meetings." She was annoyed with me. "There will always be one or two people who will say I've never been clean: I've been taking buprenorphine. I'm just addicted to another drug. They'd say I need to wake up and not use any medication. Free from all drugs is best for everyone. I don't need to hear that right now.

"Maybe I should try another meeting so I can avoid eternal damnation." She said it sarcastically to make me back off about meetings. Would her regular attendance have guaranteed abstinence?

"I thought, Maybe I'll try Vicodin just once more—is that too much to ask?"

I was disappointed because she seemed to be saying it was just one of those things that couldn't be helped. That implied she'd had so many other errors and failures, what was one more? Over the months I had come to expect that she would listen and obey—after all, I knew better about addiction. *Look at you*, I could have said, *what do you know about what you can and can't do around drugs?* I expected total loyalty from her.

"For you it *is*," I said, but I hadn't needed to. She nodded in acceptance, but her mind had shut down, eyes open. I worried that I sounded like the omnipotent parent Lucy still yearned to have around to help with her troubles. But at the same time she would reject this person as untrustworthy, not caring enough.

Abstinence was a self-imposed restriction, but I could imagine her at the wedding—the free-flowing liquor, cigar smoke, the giddy celebration of the newlyweds. At weddings, nothing in life seems banned. I was upset because her slip seemed to indicate how little I had helped. Maybe I had invented how well she was doing. Maybe I had invested her with more power than she had in an attempt *not* to reduce her to the pitiful bits of her real life. I thought of myself as a skilled professional. Perhaps I was not so skilled. I had my doubts. Her relentless struggle filled me with weariness.

She'd been hurt regularly over the years. Her life had been full of doing things she didn't want to do. Men had done stuff to her. She'd sanctioned it, but she hadn't wanted it. I imagined her cadging a few Vicodin from a man at the wedding. It was as if men, keepers of the drugs, held her hostage. She wanted them to think well of her, and she wanted them to hand over the Vicodin. Maybe she felt condemned to addiction as she was condemned to her life with men. Addicts speak about not having a choice when offered drugs.

She'd gone to the wedding—one more thing she didn't want to do.

"You only used that once at the wedding?" I asked hopefully. Every doctor who doesn't quite trust the story he or she is hearing carries a fantasy of the police procedural as shown on television. Cops are as interested in motivation and circumstances as I am, but on TV they could force the action, the admission, make the suspect do the right thing in under an hour. But I was powerless, the tone and timing of my questions were my only ammunition. I could not live their lives for them.

"Once at the wedding, and once later that night."

It occurred to me that maybe she had never wanted to quit. The past six months had been theater, a put-on, a rehearsal of convention. She had been able to stay away from Vicodin for a while because of buprenorphine, but Vicodin had always been her greatest pleasure.

"You didn't use the day after the wedding, or any other times in South Carolina?" Sometimes I asked questions as if I were forcing myself to taste something awful, and so I asked in small bites, almost unthinkingly.

"Just those two times."

Every addict can give a reason why he or she slipped—a bad husband, a sick child, a best friend visited with a few pills or a packet of heroin and couldn't be refused. Lucy made no excuses. She could have lied about her South Carolina Vicodins—they wouldn't have shown up on a urine test today if I had ordered one—but she didn't. Today she possessed a certain directness, a lack of nonsense. She seemed to have unburdened herself of something she'd held to herself for days that had produced a kind of loneliness.

I felt I needed to say something, make the usual argument in favor of sobriety, or say something reassuring so we could keep moving through the visit—"You were bound to want to use when . . . but you'll feel better when. . . ."

But I realized she wasn't here today hoping I'd make her feel better about herself. She was here because she had stopped herself after two Vicodins and she wanted to keep stopping herself. She knew if she started again, she would lose everything she'd gotten in the past months: a job, an apartment, buprenorphine, a doctor who listened, a glimpse of a clean life.

Maybe this slip was, strangely, a relief. The worst fear was now dispelled. She had caught herself and come to me with her admission. All was not lost.

Over the years I have said, or thought to say, to many addicts: there are no excuses. You are totally responsible for all your successes and failures. You have complete control of your life. Master your fate by mastering your mind. Stop yourself from thinking all those bad thoughts. There is no such thing as luck; there are no external forces directing you; only negative thinking and self-neglect. There are no hapless victims, only those who invite their own demise. Regret is unacceptable, just change your thinking and desires and you will achieve.

There remained an optimistic part of me that believed her use of Vicodin in South Carolina was an easily correctable error, a recoverable wrong turn, an aberration. I wanted her to have a smooth sail, a simple story of success, a happy ending. But there was another part of me that wanted to say to Lucy: you don't deserve my help if you can't effectively make use of it.

She would not openly apologize to me or anyone else, but she was full of remorse. How disappointed could I be with someone who blamed herself? Even as one part of me believed that the practice of medicine allowed for the profound effect people can have on one another, another part believed I hadn't helped her. What had I really offered besides a daily medication, my understanding that life was hard, and a monthly dose of optimism and benign advice? What were the right techniques or discipline I should have offered her so that she might have avoided this slip? Should I have told her that this wedding was going to be dangerous for her, and that she needed to shift her plans?

"Did you expect the visit to South Carolina—the wedding, all the time with your family—to trigger a craving for Vicodin?"

She looked at the door, thinking; how she answered seemed important to her.

"It didn't really trigger a craving. Not a craving for drugs. It triggered hopelessness. My life doesn't matter. It's already too bad to fix. I can't resolve it. It will never get better. That's when the idea of using drugs enters my brain. No, it's not about the drugs. It's just that I'm overwhelmed. It's a fight I can't win. I'm not sure what I want: to be happy, to not use drugs, to have a healthy, productive life? I get melodramatic. I start thinking I deserve to suffer for some reason and then I start to believe it. My parents think I'm okay because they've imagined I have a career in the business world.

"My mother said over and over that I seemed much better, that she felt closer to me, she wasn't as worried, she could sleep. When the doorbell rang at home she didn't think any longer that it was the police coming to tell her I'm dead. She said, 'I feel like I have a daughter again.'

"I stopped the Vicodin the morning after the wedding because I knew a week later I would be asking myself why I'd started again. On the flight back I actually felt as if there was a chance it might turn out all right, that my parents weren't going to have to watch me die."

I should have been content that during our months together she had won back some capacity for life. With the news of her slip, I needed to maintain my best hopes for her. Was the fact that she had come back to see me today enough to call the treatment a success? It was.

Outside, the sky was a dusty elephant gray, heavy with advancing rain.

"How's it been since you've been back?" I asked.

"Not good. I'm not in a good frame of mind. I feel bad for myself. I didn't want to come today. I didn't want to have to come back here. Although if I didn't come back it meant I had to use. To you it may not have meant that, but it did to me. If I walked away—I've done it enough times—I knew I would use and it would get bad, and I knew I could take it. There's no physical punishment that's too much for me.

"What should I do—keep coming or not?—that's what I've been thinking all week. I haven't wanted to talk to anyone or do anything. I've had way too much time to think. I had nothing to do in South Carolina but think about how miserable my life is, what a fucking wreck my life is.

"I look at my parents and sometimes I'm angry, but mostly I think: How the fuck did I do what I did coming out of a family like this? What happened? You and everyone else probably think the same thing. It's a good question." She stopped and laughed, which was filled with disgust for herself.

"I didn't grow up in the ghetto surrounded by people with needles in their arms. People I know look at me and are baffled: even other addicts. They can see how other people became addicts, but not me.

"I don't know what my parents think. That I just rose up out of the swamp? When I told my mother before the wedding that

I've held the same job for the past four months, she said, 'You could have done that a few years ago, you just weren't ready.' 'I think you misunderstand,' I told her. 'It wasn't a matter of not being ready. Do you understand I have a very serious illness?' 'I know. But you're better now,' she said. I told her, 'I *am* better. But just so you understand. It wasn't that I wasn't ready, or that I was lazy and didn't feel like working, or I was just a little mixed up, or some other euphemism for the past decade. Come on.' But she brushed that off, too. Maybe it sank in and she heard more than I think. It's just a really funny way of saying what happened to me. There's a lot that goes unsaid in my family. I don't know what's better: parents who keep up an unrealistic idea of who I am, or parents who write me off completely? Sometimes I wish they'd write me off."

"I've seen your good side," I said. I wanted her to know I understood that quitting was not as simple as nondrug users thought. Each visit I felt it was a struggle to reach her without making too many mistakes along the way. "Since I've known you, your life has gotten consistently better."

"I don't know if I can keep it up." She knew every day she was using Vicodin there was a more dignified way to live.

"I think you can."

"I'm still anxious from my visit with them. It's this charade of mutual lying. It's a situation where they want to pretend I am a fun, happy, whole person, and so I pretend, too. By the time I left, I could hardly breathe."

"You still feel that way?"

"Worse. Worse than I have in a long time without a doubt. I can't live with this level of fear and anxiety. I have it all the time. It's absurd. I'm afraid of too many things. You don't want me to make a list. I'm afraid of everything and its opposite. I'm afraid I'm not going to have medical care when I need it and I'm afraid of going to get it. I'm afraid of having a normal job and not having one. When I hear a sound, I jump. It doesn't take much. My heart races, the whole bit. I don't want to live like this. Even if I have the ability to accomplish something I can't concentrate. I feel like I might as well end my life or do more drugs."

I didn't believe she was suicidal, but I had to ask now that she'd brought it up. "You want to hurt yourself?"

Drug-related overdose deaths often occur in just these instances when an addict hasn't used in a long while and starts up again, returning quickly to his or her peak dose when the body isn't prepared to metabolize high levels of opiate. In such cases, opiates suppress the respiratory drive; the addict stops breathing. Vicodin users rarely overdose, as compared with heroin users, three-quarters of whom have witnessed overdoses. Few of them called ambulances, even for their friends, fearing arrest. Over half of all deaths among heroin injectors have been due to overdose. Were they suicides? Mistakes? Were these addicts so oblivious they couldn't fathom that they might die?

With Lucy, I wasn't really upset about the slip in South Carolina, but about the possibility that the two times she used would cascade and Vicodin take over her life again.

One of my other buprenorphine patients, Christina, a tough woman who worked in a doughnut shop, had recently been shaken by her best friend's overdose. Christina had used heroin with her friend for years, the two of them quitting together at the beginning of the summer. "She came over to my house last week," Christina told me at her last visit, "to invite me out. 'I've got to get it out of my system and use one more time,' Bonnie said. But I wouldn't go with her because I've been doing good with the buprenorphine. Bonnie came back about an hour later.

We were sitting in the kitchen, drinking coffee, when she put her head down and closed her eyes and her lips went blue and then her skin went gray as clay and she stopped breathing. I knew what it was. I called the ambulance and rode in the back with her to the hospital. She never said a word, never woke up on the way there, and then they wouldn't let me into the room with her because they said I wasn't family.

"I'll never forget what she looked like," Christina said, shaking her head. "She had two kids, one twenty-one, one nineteen, who I knew all their lives. The older one called me up that night and said, 'If she hadn't come to see you, she never would have done that.' I knew she was just looking for someone to blame, but I didn't let her blame me."

Watching addicts walk in and out of my office, I sometimes forget that addiction can be a fatal illness. And then I hear a story like Christina's.

One more time. To get it out of my system. Was that what it was like for Lucy in South Carolina?

"No, I'm not planning to hurt myself," Lucy said. Her reproach of me was really self-reproach. "I haven't completely lost my mind."

"You felt less afraid when you were using?"

"I don't remember. But there's some stuff I can't get rid of. The terror; I'm terrified all the time—that's not any better."

"Do you think your terror predated your drug use?"

"When I used opiates, I wasn't afraid. My dad once asked me, when I was twenty-three, I remember exactly where it was, we were on this mountaintop in Vermont, 'What is the attraction?' I told him it takes away all my fears and all my pain. He couldn't argue with that. He was silent for two minutes. He understood it existentially. I think he has the same level of anxiety."

I wondered if a happy and contented person would ever enjoy Vicodin in the same way that Lucy, Joe, and Julia did. Or was its attraction—the warmth, security, and relaxation they swore it provided—only experienced by those who moved through life without these sensations? If I were secretly slipped a Vicodin, would I find it pleasurable? Lucy's brain chemistry was undoubtedly different from mine. But her *expectations* were different, too. Knowing the next Vicodin would bring relief must have been a large part of what she enjoyed about it, and why the possibility of using again took up so much space in her mind for so many years.

"I'm not sure I can translate it," Lucy continued. "It's so big. It's waiting for me right under the surface of my life. It becomes like panic. I can't breathe. I have a physical reaction. That feeling like it would be better to jump off a building. It gets worse at times, but I'm learning that it usually doesn't kill me. It's possible to sit it out. Getting high didn't work in getting rid of it. If Vicodin took care of it even one in a hundred times, I'd still probably be using, but using didn't help."

I was surprised. For Lucy, Vicodin was obviously potent in some ways, but not in others. Was she waiting for something horrible to happen? Was she scared of Brian, who might threaten her today, tomorrow, or next week? Whoever, whatever she dreaded, she didn't want to think about it.

"Why haven't you jumped?" As soon as I heard myself I thought this was probably the wrong way to ask it, but what was the right way? If she could come up with a reason, I would be less worried.

"I thought if I had a life, a happy life, an untortured life, if only that were a possibility, my fear would go away. But I'm not sure I believe that one hundred percent. If I weren't worried about my finances, or if I could hold my head up with my family, maybe it will go away. But I'm afraid it won't and I won't get better."

If someone is depressed, to dwell on the past seems like a bad idea. There were questions I didn't want to ask Lucy, but we were near something important. "Is your fear tied to some event I don't know about? Did something happen to you?"

"I never thought so until I took out a piece of paper and made a timeline when I was in South Carolina. I thought about a cluster of events I never think about. All this stuff that happened around the same time when I was eight. Seven people in my father's family died within two years—uncles, cousins, my grandmother. I thought my fear of death and anxiety came from that, and it might have. But there were other events, too. I don't remember exactly the beginning of my anxiety and nightmares, but it all took over long before my drug days."

What happened? She must have been molested, I thought again. Probably by the father who knew her well enough to see how deep she was into drugs, who had his own notable anxiety. What else could still be affecting her life twenty years later? It was right out of a textbook—nearly half of female opiate users report sexual abuse during their childhood, and that number has to be an underestimate given the powerful reasons people don't want to admit to such horrors. It wasn't hard to convince myself this had to be right. This explained why she wasn't apologetic about her slip: drugs were the least of her problems, to her mind.

Why do I like to work with addicts? There is a hint of something familiar to me that I want or need to hear or observe. A stubbornness, a resentfulness. They have a harassed, wary, tentative way of moving through the world that resonates with me. A sense they have survived something as I had after my father died and my mother left me alone in our house night after night, working late, staying over at the houses of her friends. Like Lucy, I had a sense that life, authentic life, was supposed to be a struggle and a search for affirmation, comfort, ease, love. I looked around the office I had worked in for fifteen years. Was staying in this room a way to be protected, guarded, concealed?

When I began my medical training, I wanted to see everything. I wanted patients to bring me new problems, ones I hadn't encountered before. I believed that every patient would make me smarter, savvier, more and more satisfied with my choice of profession. Every novel clinical interaction would prime my intelligence. There was nothing duller than a solemn sameness to the day. I rooted for trouble to arrive so that I could show my stuff. I waited for the ruinous and alarming so I could take decisive action. I wasn't much interested in what happened after the patients left my office, or were discharged from the hospital. Then, after years in the presence of illness, after the sadness of too many deaths in my family, I wanted patients to bring me smaller problems, or questions I knew at least part of the answer to, that didn't require me to go to a book to feel competent. I didn't want each day to demand of me a harsh, invigorating, mind-clearing readiness to ponder new questions. Of late, I hadn't been seeking intellectual challenges at all. I wanted only the intimacy of hearing how people's lives were arranged: one parent, two grandparents, aunts coming and going, distressed and chaotic lives, Guatemalan, Russian, Cambodian lives in voices soft with the syllables of other countries, explaining what it was like to live on $600 a month for a family of four, or in a trailer, or with the heat off for a week, or without ever having bought a piece of new clothing, not even underwear, explaining why they came to see me, the infinite ways people live. A good day, a lucky day now, was one when I was moved by a patient. I wanted to hear a small story that reminded me I was involved in and morally committed to their medical lives, and that I had the license and ability to help a patient move from dire circumstances to more tolerable ones. Every doctor enjoys doing for others.

I knew it was hard for Lucy to ask for anything, so I never made her ask. I couldn't wait another month to see Lucy. I needed to assure myself this was not the beginning of a new phase, the return to daily Vicodin use and dependence. I took out my prescription pad and wrote for her usual buprenorphine dose of two pills a day, fourteen in total.

"Come back in a week. I want to hear how you're doing."

She agreed.

PART III

CHAPTER 8

Tuesday, December 24

Lucy had missed her last appointment. She had now been gone for over a month. I presumed what had happened to her was the same as what happened to Lauren, who'd relapsed ninety days into sobriety.

I'd been seeing Lauren since August. She was in her late forties with thick auburn hair, a thin silver anklet, and an inability to stay employed for very long. Just after Thanksgiving she had been laid off from her cosmetic counter job at a department store. She had a few friends who were renting ski houses. Several afternoons this month she had sat near a fireplace staring at the slopes through the window, smoking a little marijuana, eating a little salad, snorting a little cocaine, tasting some sushi, swallowing a few Vicodin—your basic winter picnic.

She claimed she had never stopped her buprenorphine, which surprised me. Taking Vicodin on top of a stable dose of buprenorphine usually produced no kick, no additional relaxation. I thought those few patients who claimed effects were imagining them, thinking back to earlier times.

This was the third time in a row Lauren had come into my office with all of these drugs appearing in her urine toxicological results. What was my plan? At her first two visits, we talked about her triggers, whether her far-too-patient husband, a former addict, knew about her relapse.

"Of course he does," Lauren confirmed lightly. "We've been married twenty-five years. 'Your voice sounds funny.' That's his way of saying it. Even my fifteen-year-old son knows. He said it in his own way, 'Why are you acting weird today, Mom?'"

Lauren and I talked about looking for new work to keep her busy. I told her that I thought she should work, if she could work. The structure of a workday kept temptation at bay. "My son says if I work at Burger King it would be too embarrassing for him— 'What if my friends come in and see you?'"

At Lauren's third visit, I told her, "If this keeps up, it's telling the two of us that buprenorphine may not be the best choice for you any longer."

I said "this" and "it's" as if somehow the relapse wasn't Lauren's doing. She had been on methadone and didn't want to go back on that. Her methadone program was behind the train tracks in her hometown, in a small white building with metal grilles on the windows set back behind low bushes that didn't seem to grow. It sat next to the county's Police Department Training Academy in a depopulated area; no residential neighborhood wanted a program and its clientele—the limping and tattooed who wore clothes that were too big or once belonged to someone else.

"I feel like you're threatening me," she said angrily. She leaned forward in her chair, puffing up her chest. "I tell you the truth about what I've been doing and you use it against me. It makes me not want to tell the truth." She tried to look hurt.

"I'm glad you tell me what's been going on, but your toxicology results tell me the truth also." I wanted to sound grateful, but uncowed. I had her trapped, the perfect conversational strategy. I could give a lecture for as long as I liked. I could chastise her until she never wanted to see me again, or until she thought I wanted to get rid of her.

"You don't think I could get around your toxicologies? You don't think I could bring in urines that would be negative? Lots of people do. Lots of people you see here do." Her insult—that I was easily duped, and worse, didn't even know I was being taken—didn't bother me; I could see how upset she was. I knew the tricks to beat the urine test as well as she did: drinking vinegar or lemon juice an hour before collection time, or adding a little bleach to the test cup.

"Don't get angry at *me*," I said. I was calm because I had always been good to Lauren. "Be angry at yourself for going backwards. I'm trying to help you, but you need to get it together again and stop using."

I told her the problem wasn't so much the marijuana, or even the cocaine (which she had dabbled in for years and about which she had heard from me a listing of every health risk associated, and there were plenty, including stroke, heart attack, and sudden death)—it was the opiates. To continue to use opiates while returning for prescriptions of buprenorphine suggested either she was willing to waste her money (unlikely), or she was not using buprenorphine so that she could have the Vicodin effect. If number two were the case, what was she doing with the buprenorphine?

Giving it to friends, selling it? This was how the black market in any valued substance continued, medications taken from perfectly valid prescriptions and put into circulation on the street.

When I told Lauren I was on the verge of discontinuing her from the program, I had morphed into another no-good doctor. I was no longer her white-coated supporter, but an enemy who was ruining her life. As if she hadn't been trying to ruin it herself for twenty years. Whatever I said next wouldn't stop her from thinking badly of me, the cruel taskmaster who was trying to blackmail her into sobriety by holding her buprenorphine hostage. She had been angry, but in the style of a good actress. Now she looked at me imploringly, her eyes teeming.

"What do you want me to do?"

"I want you to come back next week after not using anything except buprenorphine this week."

She had been on a once-a-month schedule, so this was a dramatic change. She would have fewer pills at home; she would have the additional co-pays for the extra visits; she would have to look me in the eye.

"Come back in a week? You're treating me differently from the way you treat other patients."

"Actually, I'm not." I liked Lauren, her generally good humor, her energy. But she'd also been particularly draining in the length and wildness of her excuses, her sometimes slavering need for encouragement, her sexualized, pseudo-smitten, sit-too-close focus.

She saw this change as a punishment, and it was in a way. But I worried that I had sent an inadequate message of disapproval. What lesson was I trying to impart? That I needed her to work harder? That I wanted her to do more than manage her symptoms? That I had the power to give comfort and take it away? We both knew there was little I could dictate. I might awaken her desire to change but I couldn't force it.

"A week. Because you need to get a grip on this now."

As Lauren was leaving, I remembered Julia saying to me, on her way out the door at our last visit, "Is drug abuse really a disease? I guess what I'm asking is, can it run in families? I'd rather it not be a disease. My mother would like to say it's a disease so she can get pity. I'd rather say I got lost, or I was weak. You've talked about brain scans. My mother is certain she caused damage to her brain from taking tranquilizers. But her scan was fine."

There is nothing to suggest that opiate addicts have experienced brain damage; there is nothing grossly amiss from a neurological vantage or noted in structural brain imaging. Subtler tests of brain function can uncover abnormal findings in some patients, but who is to say these didn't predate opiate use (maybe even led to opiate use), or weren't the result of one or another drug known to be toxic—nicotine, alcohol—that addicts often use.

Not only Julia, but many observers, doctors included, are uncomfortable calling opiate addiction a disease. Although dependence on opiates has a genetic inheritability and neurochemical sequelae, no one listening in on my visit with Lauren could deny there is a volitional aspect as well; her intentions couldn't be ignored. A patient's inability to control her behavior might be associated with her brain chemistry or could be pictured by a neuroimaging study, but these findings don't prove addiction is a disease. No more than physiological changes in the brain can prove hunger is a disease. Diabetes and asthma, which require medications, but also have critical behavioral components like watching one's diet or taking medications, are not questioned as diseases—is addiction analogous?

Central to addiction is loss of control, but how much has to be lost? If there are people like Monica who can use heroin in a controlled manner, do they have a disease? Not all difficult-to-control habits are called diseases. Cigarette smoking is rarely called a disease, although perhaps it could be. Economists have argued that the same principles that govern substance abuse govern consumption of other goods. Addicts are rational consumers who are motivated to maximize satisfaction (greater energy, less anxiety, an extraordinary head-rush experience) under conditions of constraint on access (price, risk of arrest, risk of exposure, alternative behavior choices). Loss of control implies loss of free will, and Lauren had plenty of will. To say she didn't would diminish her responsibility.

I wanted Lauren to regain the sense of responsibility she'd shown increasingly over the last months, but seemed to have lost when she was laid off. But if addiction was an uncontrollable disease, how could I expect Lauren to control herself? I didn't expect my patients with multiple sclerosis to control their symptoms.

Lauren missed her next appointment, my last appointment of the week the previous Friday. I sat at my desk waiting. I waited long enough to realize she wouldn't be back.

Lucy called to get on my schedule on the day before Christmas. She had been gone for almost five weeks. She had presumably run out of the fourteen buprenorphine tablets from her last prescription weeks before, which meant she had returned to opiates. Her slip had become a full-fledged relapse.

Why had Lucy relapsed? Like every doctor caring for addicts, I was hungry for a test that could distinguish those at risk for relapse from those who weren't. I was eager to replace the standard mode of prediction—questionnaires of life history and life context factors, a checklist of relapse risks such as unemployment, few supportive friends, nonparticipation in NA. I wanted a brain scan—that science fiction trope that for a decade had appeared in scientific journals and newspaper articles in dazzling shades of emerald, yellow, and red that supposedly represented the activities of both consciousness and unconsciousness—that could literally "read a person's mind." I was as technology besotted as the next person, but there was no evidence that these scans were useful for such predictions yet. The craving region of the brain was not small. Could the same neuronal regions activated by narcotic craving be activated by many different circumstances unrelated to drugs (skydiving? stealing?) that had equal emotional value? Were all forms of craving the same? What if the craver was taking buprenorphine, or had depression, or had suffered a past brain injury, would these affect the scan? What if a person tried not to crave during the scanning? How meaningful could a scan be that recorded a split second of neuronal action if true craving was more than momentary?

After telling me at her last visit that she had slipped at the wedding, I thought Lucy would either have to ask for help when the agonizing desire struck, or she would have to find some way of dealing with it alone. The desire to get high in the days to weeks after a slip would be so horrible, I knew, that she would pray for her head to explode. She wouldn't want those craving thoughts to stay in her mind. But she would also know that it didn't matter what she thought or believed, all that mattered was what she did. This was predicated on the belief that if she did the right things for long enough, her desires would eventually change.

What was a satisfactory outcome for Vicodin addicts in general and for Lucy Fields in particular? Was the only acceptable outcome abstinence? Or was it long-term employment (even if that required the occasional Vicodin), the satisfaction of a day's effort and the possibility of escape from poverty? Was it happiness? Was it general improvement across a variety of life domains—family, psychological, relations with men—or dramatic progress in just one of these? Would my answer be the same as Lucy's?

When I went out to get her, I saw Lucy move warily through

the waiting area, quick and fearful as though she might be stopped and questioned. I didn't want to feel an aversion, but I did. I had the sense there was nothing promising ahead. I assumed she had more bad news, and I would again be the voice of disapproval. It was amazing that all my drug-dependent patients didn't hate my guts. Maybe they did.

Of course she never sat straight, feet planted in front of her on the floor, spine to chair back. She sat askew, sideways, with her legs slung over one arm of the chair, fitting herself across her seat, shoulders hunched, trying to look comfortable, but squeezed in uncomfortably. Lucy appeared nervous; she was interested in her nails.

I dreaded this moment when I would be forced to push my authority and make demands.

"You don't have your coffee with you today," I began.

"I've already had too much," she answered. "I don't like being uncomfortable from too much caffeine. Any physical discomfort and I think I'm in withdrawal. If I'm cold or flushed or have a stomachache, my head goes immediately to withdrawal." Veins engorged on her forehead when she laughed. "I know it's not true, but I have to tell myself I'm being ridiculous."

"Tell me what happened," I said.

"For like a week after our last appointment, I thought about taking Vicodin. I'd had an awful feeling that week, this feeling that I was forgetting something. Like there was something I should feel horrible about, but couldn't remember it. This all-over body feeling, that took over my arms, my legs. I woke up feeling that way and it went all day.

"Then one day I saw this kid I knew from being with Brian, and he said, 'Could you give me a ride?' It was lunchtime and Marie had lent me her car so I could run an errand or two during my break. She's been really nice to me since the whole Luther thing.

This kid gets in the car and the first thing he says is, 'So what do you want?' And I answer, 'Are there any cheap Vics around?' 'I'll see,' he says, and he gets on his phone and starts speaking Spanish. He hangs up and says, 'Let's go over near the hospital to pick it up.' 'I'm not going there,' I said. That was too much for me, picking up drugs right outside the building where I come to see you. He gets back on the phone. He finds another guy who's at a McDonald's across town. We start driving there. Within two minutes, he starts talking sexual stuff. Very graphically about some women he had sex with. I pull over. I back the car into this space and as I'm doing it, I hit the car behind me, just enough to jar me. Part of my mind clicks on. It was as if I'd forgotten that whole aspect, the whole element of having to listen to and put up with this kind of shit. I get out to see if I scratched Marie's car, and he gets out and says, 'What, what?' 'I'm not sure I want to use,' I tell him. There was no scratch. 'You think about it,' he says, and walks away. He comes back five minutes later and hands me one hundred pills.

"I had time to change my mind, but I didn't," Lucy said.

"You reentered your old life," I said.

"I forget how easy it was."

"Did you know when you saw him where all this was headed?"

"I must have. I'd seen him before, and I kept going back."

"Weren't you scared of letting him into the car?"

"I'm not scared of the right people. Which is pretty strange, because I'm scared of everything and everyone pretty much. But not him on a day when I felt ready to use."

Hearing this brought a sinking sensation. "And then?"

"I used the hundred pills in ten days."

Had she lost her job? Gone back to Brian for the next hundred pills? I wondered about her list of what she needed to do on a day when she was using. Go to the bank, get coffee, get library card, walk to mall, buy Vicodin.

"I reached a point where either I had to go forward and accept having a life that's all right, or go back to drugs full-time. You'd think it's a no-brainer, but it's not. I feel like I have to make that decision all the time actually, and most days I'm on the fence."

Listening is a terrible business, almost impossible to manage at times. Lucy's story was painful to listen to: one doesn't elect to be an addict.

"What about today?"

"I went back on the buprenorphine after the Vicodin ran out, using the pills I had left over, putting myself through the withdrawal you did with me eight months ago.

"Let me describe the ways I've ruined my life," Lucy continued. "I had ability and potential, but I've chosen to be a loser. I'm fucking pathetic. I've squandered my life and opportunities. Pretty much that's the way it looks to me. After doing shit for ten years, I will never get to do what I might have wanted to.

"Not only did I lose part of my life, but also the only identity I ever had. I have no purpose. I'm floating around. At least when I was an addict I knew what I was going to do in the morning and why I needed to do it.

"I'm not sure I can deal with it, this complete devastation that is my life."

"But you have dealt with it. You've gotten your own place to live. You've held a job."

She didn't correct me. "I have to stop myself from thinking too much. Five minutes by myself is too much. If I go out somewhere and forget to bring my book, I'm lost. I'm very uncomfortable. If I'm not constantly occupied, then I'm left to myself, and I do things like go to where I'll run into that kid."

I knew she needed a solid life structure, but I hadn't realized that even the smallest opening in her daily calendar was hard to contend with, too easy to fill with bad times.

"When I pass that place, I feel so ashamed," she said. "You know that expression 'burning shame'? That's the feeling I have: hot, flushed."

"What are you ashamed of?" I was ready to hear Lucy apply the usual rant about addicts—they were depraved, defective, immoral—to herself.

"I'm ashamed I could take down all I've built in one day. I'm ashamed that I made up a fake life, a life that appeared normal, eight months ago. People at Pets Plus know a *part* of my real life, but no one else knows any of it. Maybe everyone puts up a fake front so death doesn't chase them."

Was she scared that death was chasing her? More than once she'd told me she didn't believe in God or daily miracles or blessing or sin or the mysteries of the universe. She was a pragmatist. Maybe her dread and anxiety were existential.

"It looks like I'm going back to school," she said. She said it without emotion. Outside, I noticed easy clouds, a mild wind, and the visible breath of people on the street.

"You are?" I was dumbfounded. After her relapse, some part of me expected her life to be one of sorrow without conclusion.

"I have a financial aid meeting over at the state college tomorrow. I have thirteen thousand in loans from my earlier education lying in a heap of dust. I had forbearance on those loans, but I probably need to pay off about $1,500 to get a new loan. That degree was useless, even though it was from a good school. I was semiconscious during the whole thing. I have no idea how I got the degree that I did. But it was so long ago I decided I have to go back and take a few undergrad courses to move ahead, like if I want to get a master's degree in something. I can't get recommendations from my old school. That was ten years ago, too long ago even if I *had* good relationships with any professors. I don't even know if they still teach or if they'd remember me. To study for

GREs would take a year, so I might as well go back. I still don't know what I want to study in graduate school."

I was stunned. Graduate school?

"The state school is only like two thousand dollars a semester. It's a pretty good deal, and new classes start in a couple of weeks. I have to do something. I can't work jobs like the one I have indefinitely. It's driving me mad; I need to cut back at the pet store. Marie has been vicious, off-and-on cruel, looking for things I do wrong, tiny irrelevant things. I think when I told her that I was going to school again, I suddenly became just too successful for her. She whispers with the drunk woman and the personality-disordered girl when I come into the room now. I left her a note apologizing that my school schedule is still unclear, that the only day I can commit to after Christmas is Saturday, and I think that's what set her off. Plus, they're going out of business, I think. I can't put myself in the position of having no work. I can't earn enough money there to get along. I have to go to school to get back to where I should be, or where my parents think I should be."

Was all this good news a misdirection, a distraction? Was telling me this a way of avoiding the continuing Vicodin use or was she trying to demonstrate to me that life could proceed even with a little narcotic in one's system?

"If it makes your parents so happy, maybe they should pay for school," I suggested, smiling. I was thinking about the tuition payments I had set aside for my college-bound son. Lucy was dressed like a student in a white long-sleeved cotton shirt. She wore hole-in-the-knee jeans, white socks, and heeled, black clogs. She had two silver necklaces, two small hoops in her right ear, and a plain gold ring on her left middle finger.

"I actually called my mother and told her I filled out all the school forms and sent in a $500 first installment for classes. If I act like I'm expected to, my parents like it. Going to school is the only way to make my family happy. For almost ten years my father has been offering me money for tuition as an inducement to go to school. They're pushing me to take their money: it's degrading, insulting. Of course it's also humiliating. It's a way of saying, 'You are not who you should be by now.' The implication is: not like your sister. She has a Lexus. Of course it came with her husband. She married a Lexus.

"I was thinking I could tell my father I was going to school, take his money, put it into savings, have a little cushion, and put off classes for a while. Part of me says he owes me. And part of me says I don't want any more obligations to them."

"When did all this happen?"

"Right before I went to South Carolina, I went over to the college to meet someone from the admissions office. I didn't want another BA, but there were advantages to matriculating rather than just auditing—health insurance, financial aid. The admissions woman said if I did a year, then I could finish my prerequisites for most graduate programs. I've been thinking of getting a psychology degree, maybe work as a youth counselor. It was strange to be talking about actually starting school in a month.

"I expected it to fall through. It was really strange making plans. It had been such a long time since I did anything productive or had success at something. Strange. As of Friday, I have three letters from the school tacked to the bulletin board in my apartment. A letter congratulating me on my admission. Another letter saying they're pleased to offer me aid. And a third saying something else. It's the first time I've felt wanted. And they made it happen so fast."

"Feels good, doesn't it?"

"Yeah, but alien, and a little slick. I feel like I'm an imposter.

Cleverly concealed. To have a plan is weird. I'm used to sitting around and talking about things I'd do some day. Detox, get a new apartment, a new job, travel. I'll do them all tomorrow. It's strange that it's actually happening. I feel like it will evaporate. I'll wake up and it won't be there. It was all a junkie delusion. But I'm ready to go back to school, if only to hold my head up."

This change for Lucy was late arriving, but not impossible. Two weeks after relapsing had she rediscovered self-regulation? I wondered how, after a decade and a half of lies, fears, and pains, she could fathom normalcy. School, a better job, money in the bank—it must have felt like a ruse, a trick, a trapdoor. It was terrifying, and she already lived surrounded by fears. But I also knew she was angry at herself for wasting time, ten years of it.

Three thousand days and nights of opiates circulating in your body are not easily set aside, and she had relapsed. Today, the tension of needing to use again did not seem to be building in her. One had to respect the past, the power of it, the years of fervor and passion of the wrong kind. Some patients need contact with that past, reaching back before leaving it.

"Are you still working at Pets Plus?" I asked.

"Yes, I am," she answered firmly. "I need the money. I actually sort of like working there. I was thinking the other day about when I was twenty-one and just done with college and my Vicodin use was really picking up. I was sleeping in my parents' basement and living off Pixy Stix and peanut butter cups. They had a dog they pretty much ignored. And he would visit me and we became friends, maybe because I fed him candy. I really couldn't love anything at that point, but when their terrier came downstairs, it was the first time I recall having had a feeling for a living thing. I looked forward to seeing him. It must have been a crack in the ice—not like it lasted. Before him and after him I had no feelings, or none that I could process. Anyway, there's a dog at the shop now who looks like Scamper."

"You know I have to ask this," I said. I was happiest when drugs were not the pretext, context, and subtext of every minute of every visit.

She was prepared for the question and I didn't even need to finish. "None. Nothing in a week. I have no Vicodin in my apartment. Gone." She said it with a sweet, insinuating emphasis.

Hesitantly, I made myself smile. I smiled at the luck of it. It seemed as if, in a week, she'd put better times in motion on her own. My optimistic outlook returned.

"Not that I don't have reason to use." Her voice was flat, without any grief or anger.

"What's that?" She seemed scared. As quickly as I had become sanguine, I felt my mood dropping.

"I'm leaning toward having sex with my landlord. Why not? Am I really worth more than a few hundred dollars? I don't think I've given you a clear picture of how much pressure he puts on me. He calls me on the phone regularly. I actually asked him last time, 'Why *me*? Why are you calling me?' He said, 'You're pretty and smart and vulnerable.' Aha. There it is. Why shouldn't I have sex with him? It's not like I have dignity and value myself. I know I'm supposed to, but I don't. Part of me is like, if that's what you want, go ahead. I also know there are lots of reasons not to. It would be acting like a whore."

I was as stunned to hear this as I had been ten minutes before when I learned she was returning to school. Sometimes I zone out when patients speak. For a moment or two I get lost in a reverie about what my sons are doing at just that second, or about wildfires I'd heard about on the news, or I find myself trying to recall the name of a piece of music I'd heard on the radio on the way to work.

But I was concentrating with Lucy today; it was coming at me too fast, all the surprises and contradictions, the ups and downs.

"I know that if I act like I have dignity, one day it will be true. I also know I might be starting something here I can't get out of. It's a version of the situation I've been in my whole fucking life. I sleep with people not because I want to, but because I have to for my habit, or because they say I should. I don't want to sleep with anyone ever again."

I was stuck on her line, "acting like a whore." Had she ever sold herself, as she was implying she might with her landlord?

Her troubles with men had hovered over our conversations for months, lingered in the atmosphere, though neither of us mentioned it much. I wondered if this cloud was part of the reason I had never examined her, never even touched her, since her initial exam months before when she was in withdrawal. The more I spoke with her about intimate parts of her life, the more awkward it seemed to perform the usual maneuvers of a medical visit, the blood pressure check, placing my stethoscope to her back. My visits with Lucy did not even include a handshake; it was odd to consider that there was no contact between us whatsoever. The same was true of my visits with Julia and Lauren and Tom and Monica, so unlike the appointments of most of my patients. Most people I see offer purely physical problems—a sore elbow, a swollen toe, shortness of breath—which I examine ruthlessly for a cause, categorizing, making lists.

Because most of my general medical patients are elderly, I spend hours each day doing physicals. Every patient tips away when being scrutinized, just before I touch them. They rub their noses, shake their wrists, hide their chins in palms in an expert repertoire of self-protection. I start at the top, studying the forehead suddenly tightened by a wince, the wet eyes, the tiny bubbles at the corners of the lips, the thrumming at the base of the throat.

My older patients take slow and deep breaths. I think of their lungs as lilac bushes, a thousand purple fists opening and closing. Their legs draw up defensively. Hands drag in misgiving and regret. Age pushes itself to the surface in dry and brown spots, fibrous buttons and contracted skin. Wedding bands are buried in the flesh. At shoulders and hips and knees, bones feel like metal. Abdomens are shallow and shaky when I press. Beneath, there are parts that have outlived their usefulness. Inspecting the genitals is like picking through the ruins, a salvaging expedition. I study the underwater movements of their legs, dangling. I note a slight change in temperature as I move to the feet. Feet that were once loose and happy and new are now merely conciliatory. Their bodies speak even when their mouths don't tell the whole story.

On the other hand, addicts become tellers of stories and not bodies in the room. Young, generally healthy, they don't offer the spectacle of physical aberration. They are a different kind of enigma waiting to be solved. Each is an exercise in narrative history. Lucy would pull herself onto the small place of her chair and talk—I couldn't imagine her ever standing and stretching her arms to relax.

"Have you ever enjoyed sex?" I asked.

"Nope. Never. So why not get something for it? Money, rent. I've done enough of it without getting money."

Lucy looked preoccupied talking about sex. I thought of Lauren, who enjoyed talking about nothing more, whose affair (and lying to her recently sober husband about going to NA meetings when she was really meeting her lover) was the secret driving her back to drugs, she confided. She didn't recognize what she was about to lose. Lauren had two habits: Vicodin and self-delusion.

"It would be seedy and perverted to involve myself with him. Just my kind of thing," Lucy said meanly. "But really it's a step up from the usual people I'm with. He's decent looking, he has money—so what if he has three children? He's not a junkie or drug dealer.

"I know people say there is such a thing as a good relationship, but I doubt there's ever sex without exploitation. I'm really not sure there is."

Usually, I quieted myself, got myself out of the way when Lucy spoke. But I believed my job with her had moved beyond relief of physical or mental suffering. My job was to help her decide on appropriate actions. She was full of self-loathing.

"You know what the right thing to do here is," I insisted, more instructive than usual. Was there really a dilemma, an uncertainty, about what she should do about her landlord? She seemed to understand perfectly. Was she so turned around by her years with Brian or whomever to believe she could entangle herself with her scumbag property owner? I felt paternal. "I understand you might be worried that if you refuse, it's possible he could ask you to move out, but you could probably sue him. You should tell your roommates what's happening, so you have some allies."

"He's not threatening me. He's just persistent. I'm not happy when I see his number on my cell phone. 'I just wanted to see how you were doing,' he says. The conversation inevitably turns lewd. He has a 'job' for me if I'm interested. Everything is about sex. I'm afraid to pay him a day late. It all comes back to: Why me? Why did he pick me out? Am I doing something?"

She didn't trust herself. She didn't want a mess with her landlord; she didn't want to lose her apartment. She was trying to make an involvement with him sound logical, but really she was scared and lonely. Her behavior was out of my control, but I needed to be explicit.

"You need to stop taking his calls. You're an expert at not answering the phone at work. If you run into him, you need to tell him to leave you alone. You're engaging him. He thinks you're flirting in some way."

I felt myself getting angry at him, and at her. I heard myself talking less kindly. She knew to take precautions, to make provisions, to watch out.

"I think I probably encouraged him. I didn't do or say anything initially. He just threw out his line to see what he would get, and from me he got mixed messages, so he kept going. It's me. I'm probably not so subtle. My mother used to scream at me, 'Are you stupid?' when she saw the men who came for me.

"I could ignore his calls and send my money through my roommates, I suppose. I can't even tell the guy off. I don't say, 'Stop it,' or 'I'll call your wife.' She'd probably believe me because she probably already knows what he's like.

"I don't know why I don't just tell him 'No' and hold my ground. But I can't with people like him." She cleared her throat and sat up with a blurred look, blinking at the back of my door. She rubbed her ears with her fingers as if they were cold.

"I don't believe that." Outside my office the world is wild. I have never gotten used to the stories of how quickly addicts go into nosedives, lose everything, houses, savings accounts, jobs, spouses. Lucy was adept at losing everything.

"He's not the only one, you know. It goes on and on and on. This guy I had a relationship with four years ago. He's an older guy. He had two kids who were close to my age. He happened to come into where I work a few months ago. The next week he came back and bought me a loaf of bread. The next week he brought me bread, olives, butter, feta cheese, a thirty-dollar bag of groceries. I like food, but I can buy my own. I do everything else on my own. I can buy groceries. It's a joke at my work. 'One of Lucy's boyfriends is out front again,' I'll hear. I'm starting to realize it's ridiculous. The unacceptable behavior I put up with is getting obvious. No one else who works at Pets Plus has that kind of person coming in harassing *them*. Nobody. Luckily they think it's funny and not grounds for firing me. The guys who come in to the store these days are not even active users; the ones who are using disappeared months ago when they saw I couldn't help them. The guy with the bread was hinting that he'd bought a new house, was divorced, and maybe we should move in together.

"It's not fucking normal." She'd raised her voice, as if she were giving herself a stern lecture. "You just don't accept groceries from men. There's something wrong there. My inability to say 'Leave me alone' is not good. Before, I just saw it as part of the way I lived. I was manipulative with people. I took what I could get. That was part of my game. Even last week I took the groceries and bread. That's not good. But the scarier prospect is not standing up for myself. And continuing to be self-destructive. I can't carry on the rest of my life being afraid of people."

She had worked herself up. Listening to herself made her unhappy. Vicodin had been the old, safe context. Using a hundred pills a week allowed her to reject or deny problems such as a man bribing her into bed with bread.

I thought of Monica telling me over and over that addiction was a love affair. A special kind of love affair, she used to say, where your lover never abandoned you. If you walked out, this special lover would always take you back. He wouldn't hurt you, but he would let you hurt yourself by becoming too attached. Heroin was a lover who produced the same reliable feeling every time, one you couldn't find anywhere else, with anyone else, she said. You knew what to expect, but you carried within you your own betrayal.

"Your history has a long tail," I said to Lucy.

"I think I should get out of this city, this state. I've lived here all my life and the only people I know are addicts. I'm lonely here. It wouldn't be worse anywhere else."

Most of the Vicodin addicts I care for take their pills when they are by themselves. Taking pills isn't a social act like heavy drinking sometimes pretends to be. It lacks the paraphernalia-sharing rituals of heroin injection. Taking Vicodin was secret for Julia, Lauren, and Joe, and therefore lonely. Some of my patients are reclusive—they are big readers, TV watchers, or divorced—before they start using. Vicodin just emphasizes that one doesn't need conversation or emotional interchange to find peace.

"Have you heard from Brian?" I imagined he had somehow heard about her relapse and reappeared.

"Actually, I'm surprised he hasn't found me. I don't think he knows where I work. I moved on pretty fast."

"Any temptation to see him again?"

"No, and that's good, although I've thought about the pull of that lifestyle." She sighed. "I fear, even if I don't go back to him, I won't do a hell of a lot better. But then I think: I don't even care if I do better as long as I have my freedom."

"Maybe you see him differently now that you're clearheaded."

"*Am* I more clearheaded? I almost feel worse. Sometimes I wish I'd take the slide into complete madness. My mind manages to cling to reality, which is a fucking curse.

"My roommate was telling me the other night about how she broke up with her first love, her boyfriend of four years, and I didn't know what she even meant. I had no idea what she was feeling."

Lucy looked befuddled. I believed she had never been in love, and I thought again about Monica's description of heroin as a lover. What Lucy had been after, when she started flirting with opiates, was a feeling. It must have been a good feeling, unfamiliar at first, but one she must have felt grateful for and had to explore. Like love, opiate use must have felt so elemental it was beyond any choosing.

No wonder addicts drew me in. I invest them with myth and

romance one day, even knowing that the next day, when one stands in my doorway, back from the dead after a month or a year away, there will be nothing romantic about the official report of cruelty and deception I will hear. I am interested in love's heed-lessness, but I also know the ruinous course of its effects.

"You have a job, and now you have school plans."

"I'm exhausted. My mind is exhausted." She had a melancholy and questioning voice. She seemed to gather gloom toward her.

I knew no way to ease her mind.

"Rethinking the same shit over and over. Numbers. Combi-nations to locks. The same three-digits lock combination I've re-membered since seventh grade. The combination to my lock at the Y when I worked there for two weeks. The security code from a job I had five years ago. Letters. Words. I do it, I guess, so I don't have to think. It's a way of shutting myself off."

I thought about all the times over the past months when her eyes, turned to the door, took on a glazed look and her lips moved with an interior monologue. I wondered if she had been counting to herself. Addiction as a compulsion; she was obsessive in other ways it seemed.

"There are other things I think about that I don't want to say. Why should I reveal every last embarrassing bit of my life? Does everyone have to do that when they come in here?"

With my addicted patients in particular, I often feel close to life in flux, and I can live vicariously. They come to me having been through an ordeal and are about to embark on another. I surround myself with addicts; this must be what I want. Sometimes I know all I need to about them in a moment, sometimes I can't answer anything definitively about their character after a year with them. Each is a Rorschach, a blur of hope and disappointment, a tangled reality with no clarity to be had.

CHAPTER 9

Wednesday, February 17

In my office, patients grip the arms of their chairs like airplane
passengers in turbulence. The addicts hang on the tightest.

I'd recently seen Julia, who was filled with worries. She
had been clean for more than a year. She wore a gray turtleneck
sweater and black pants. She began the visit, as she did each one,
by smiling and saying, "I'm good," but it was quickly clear she
wasn't feeling better at all. Sometime unhappiness is like a buzz
just beyond hearing. She bit her top lip, pulling it into her mouth.
I'd asked how things were with her husband and tears came to
her dark eyes.

"It's just not in me to confide," she reported. "He always asks
about my day, and how I'm doing. I tell him about how it went,

and about our daughters when he comes in. But there are things I wish I could express that would relieve me. But I just don't. Like for the longest time I was afraid I'd get arrested. I want to tell him how that feeling started near the time I came in here, when I was still using, but it persisted after I started with you. I had the same nightmare three times a week. I was being taken away and I had seconds to say good-bye to my daughters and him. I had it again last week for the first time in a long time. I finally came out and told my husband about how this fear comes back in the evenings and he laughed. I guess he wanted to reassure me that it was ridiculous.

"My husband would like the old me back, the person he married. He saw me as a strong person. He doesn't understand where all these problems came from. He wants to blame himself—did he bring on stress that made me start using drugs? Of course he didn't. At first, I blamed motherhood. It was hectic to take care of a business and two children. Drugs helped get it done. Then I blamed it on the stress of my sister's illness. Somewhere along the way I became weak. I broke down and something got the better of me. But people see me still in a way I'm not. They see me as a strong, independent person and it's like I'm lying to them."

Julia had learned about secrecy and concealment during her childhood. Hiding was natural. Having practiced for a lifetime, she was adept at repressing certain feelings. She was filled with guilt about failing to act in time to stop her Vicodin addiction, and about her failure to speak of it later.

"My husband always asks how I am, how my doctor's appointment went. He's seen me pull it together at work over the last twelve months. I planned that birthday party for my father that went smoothly. He's seen good things. But the guilt distances me—him not knowing things. It would hurt him to know certain things—like the truth about my family. Like that my parents didn't know how to handle stress and how both of them used substances to get through and then showed that to me and my sisters. All he knows is that my mother never touched a drop of alcohol. He doesn't know she was hysterical, worried that one of us was always on the verge of dying. He doesn't know she blames her pills on what she had to go through with us, my sister's headaches, my headaches. 'You can't compare me to other mothers,' she says. No one had it worse than her. She still has her little pharmacy thing going; she's constantly in the bathroom taking things. I look at my mother and wonder what she's doing. When it came out that I had a problem with pills, she wasn't exactly judging me, but she had a look that said, 'It's okay.' Like she had something on me now.

"Will I ever get over this?" she asked plaintively. Julia was filled with sadness and regret and hollowness that must have felt like anger when she let it.

"That's what you're doing here," I said. She hadn't used Vicodin in fourteen months, but she remained racked by guilt.

"I'd like to put it all behind me and be strong again and closer to my husband. I don't want it like this for the next thirty years. He wants another child someday. But I have to be a different person to handle that and I'd have to stop the pills you give me."

After Julia got her children asleep and finished her housework, she sat in her room for an hour to "unwind." She still reported that she could take a deep breath only after she climbed into bed. Yet she told me that in general she was happier now that she was taking her medications—her buprenorphine and an antidepressant. During the past several visits she had discussed the possibility of coming off buprenorphine. Like most patients, she'd never intended to stay on it forever; she had seen it as a temporary means of regaining control over her runaway need for opiates. I'd told her at our first visit that I rarely recommended patients stop buprenorphine before six months because it always took at least that long to reorganize one's life. For patients who'd spent years using Vicodin or OxyContin or heroin, whose brain chemistry had changed in meaningful and perhaps permanent ways, I suggested far longer treatment. But I also told Julia I was completely in favor of her halting buprenorphine as soon as possible, and that I'd had plenty of patients who had successfully come off it and maintained sobriety.

I sometimes imagine sitting around one table with all the patients I've ever treated with buprenorphine. What would I toast to as I raised my glass of alcohol-free beer? To patience.

When I first hand out the buprenorphine, many patients ask, "How long do I have to take this stuff?" They want to know what the rules are. How long do they have to be good? They want me to know that if it doesn't work the way they want it to, they will leave and not come back.

Lucy had never asked about getting off buprenorphine. She had spent fifteen years as a prisoner of pills, and she was having a hard time getting over her past. She knew that in our months together she had never been far from relapse. She also understood the perilous truth that stopping buprenorphine would send her through less severe withdrawal than coming off Vicodin, but an uncomfortable one nonetheless. I had taken many patients off buprenorphine, gradually lowering their doses until it was gone. But Lucy had used pills since she was a girl; a life without any pills was unimaginable.

Julia was not sure she should stop buprenorphine and raised the idea tentatively. I was uncertain, too. The uncertainty I offer patients is a sign of good faith. If she stopped buprenorphine, did that mean she was "better"? Drug addiction isn't a urinary tract infection where doctor and patient can be sure it is cured because the burning sensation resolves; it isn't gout, time limited and relieved with an anti-inflammatory agent, the swelling and redness gone.

Addiction is different. I am never sure when it is over; many addicts are sure it is never over. As a disease, it isn't like gout or even hypertension, which is silent in a patient's body until its unmistakable consequences become clear. As a mental illness (to a great degree public health groups and insurers accept its full disease status), addiction is chronic, intermittently intrusive, or overwhelming. But addiction is the only disease it is illegal to have. It is the only disease you can be jailed for. If I reject the disease model (as Julia wanted to), then my role is not curative, but is instead a matter of setting limits and rules, of offering rewards (fewer visits with me) and expectations, of threatening with sanctions (being denied further buprenorphine or asked not to return) until a patient's "strength" revives. But is discharging a patient who isn't violent or abusive to me or my staff ever defensible when I know that the consequences (overdose, imprisonment, HIV infection) can be catastrophic? I want patients to exercise restraint around drugs, just as I want them to exercise as a way of reducing their blood pressure and losing weight. I have come to believe that it doesn't matter if opiate dependence is a disease; what matters is that it's lethal.

When Julia had begun therapy, I believed that she was a good candidate to finish buprenorphine within the year. She had used opiates for a relatively brief time. But when I asked her at her most recent visit how she would handle stress in the future without buprenorphine, she said, "I never had a way before and I don't know what I'd do now. But I'm worried my husband is getting impatient. There's a change in his tone, like, 'I'm not even going to ask you anymore what's going on.' I know he feels distant."

"How do you know?"

"I hear him on the phone. He used to mention my name a lot when he spoke to friends. He was proud of me. When things were going well at work for me, it made him so happy. Now I don't hear him say my name hardly at all when he's on the phone."

Six months after I'd referred Marco to methadone treatment because of his inability to become abstinent under my care, he reappeared in my office. Without his chef's tunic, he looked smaller. He wore loose jeans and a checkered button-down and cowboy boots.

"I ran into some trouble," he said.

Marco had seemed impatient and incautious in the past, but he was a little humbler now; he spoke more slowly. I remembered feeling, when he was with me before, that I had tried harder than he had to get him healthy. His kitchen coworkers always had pills for him and he had accepted their offers; he hadn't worked to find a group of sober friends.

"What kind of trouble?"

"I got arrested for having Xanax on me. I'm going to court again next week."

"I'm not following you," I said. "Why did you get arrested for Xanax?" A legal tranquilizer that has addictive potential, Xanax is not a favorite medication of mine for calming the anxieties of opiate-dependent patients, but having a few shouldn't put a person in jail.

"I was over at the house of this guy who lives on my street. His house was obviously under surveillance. There were visitors going in and out all day, I didn't know any of them, and the state police came in and arrested the house owner and another guy who was supposedly on parole for armed robbery. I was there so they took me, too, and I had one Xanax pill on me because I always carry around one. When I told them I had a prescription, they said, 'You can tell the judge.' The police weren't looking for me and so it shouldn't be a problem in court."

The story didn't quite make sense to me, but I often hear things from addicts that don't sound right. One day Marco was a chef, the next he was in jail? Many addicts are petty criminals, or hang around with people on parole or probation. They peacefully recast relationships and incidents from their lives when they want something from me. They have ingenious ways to frame their troubles. But I am just as capable of double-talk, maneuvering, and delays when I want to hold something back. I can censor my personality as they can.

"What about opiates?" I asked. "You were considering methadone when I last saw you."

"Yeah. I didn't go. I had some pills left over from the last prescription you'd given me, and I cut them in half for a while. Then I didn't take anything for a while. Then I went back on OxyContin, and then I stopped that, too."

"You were able to stop on your own?"

"I didn't sleep for forty-eight hours, and then just a little for about five more days. I was clean except for the Xanax that I got from another doctor to help me with sleep. When I got arrested, my wife threw me out and I went to live with my parents who said I should get into a program."

"You have any more Xanax around?" I asked. I'd never liked Marco, but I admired his assertiveness. I remembered finding him intimidating, not threatening, but in a more pointed way: he didn't care what I thought. He refused to accept my advice.

"I gave the bottle to my lawyer. I've pretty much locked myself into my parents' house so I don't run into anyone and I'm clean if the judge asks for a urine."

"You're not on OxyContin now?"

"I went for a while without it and I see what that's like now. Four weeks off, that's the longest it's been in six years. But to be honest, I couldn't tell you I won't take any Oxy for the rest of my life. I can picture myself taking it again. That's why I need buprenorphine, because I don't want to go back."

Before your court date, I thought to myself. Sometimes the risk of incarceration is enough to scare people away for a few years. Obviously Marco's OxyContin use would come up in court, and if he was in treatment, his parents were right, it would serve his legal defense.

"Work?" I asked.

"I assume they'll take me back. I'm suspended right now. It seems like I'm in trouble, but really I'm not—I had a prescription."

He cast his Xanax use as a misstep, something minor. But it was not insignificant, and I knew we'd be talking more about it after he cleared his court case. I gave Marco a prescription for enough buprenorphine for a week. I believe in second chances, and usually third chances as well.

Lucy came in energetically. Certain aspects of the woman I'd met ten months ago were mostly gone, her weariness, her slackness. She was wearing jeans, and a blue vest over a black shirt. Her sneakers were purple, with orange socks. She laid a Jane Smiley paperback on the floor next to her coffee and took out a mortarboard. I had seen Lucy once in January, and she was doing well. She was "trying to be a halfway responsible person, like communicating with my mother and father and sister." She'd had another drug-free month confirmed by a toxicological test.

"How's school?" I asked.

"I'm taking two classes. One is this writing class. It has two men and about fifteen women. At the first class people went around the room introducing themselves and telling what they've been doing over the past five years. They all told their stories. One had a kid. One got married. One got his black belt in karate."

"What did you say?"

"I said I got a degree and worked for a couple of years. Not exactly true. Not to be snotty, but no one went to a school of the caliber that I did. I have credentials even if they're a little out-dated. On the other hand, I don't even have a computer.

"I've written one paper. It seemed pretty nonacademic to me. The assignment was to tell about a time you helped someone. I figured it was confidential, so I wrote about helping a girl I knew when I was waitressing who was in a drug treatment program. I haven't really helped anyone else. Addiction was the only thing that popped into my mind for the essay. It made me think: Do I really even *have* other experiences outside of substance abuse? I had two pages, double-spaced, what could I say? I took the girl to meetings; I talked to her on the phone. Nothing amazing. She relapsed anyway."

Lucy was unsentimental. Listening, I wondered if I had in-vented her—was she meaner and colder than I realized?

"The next week the professor asked me to read it out loud. One of the two guys in the class, he must be twenty-one years old, says, 'There are certain people you can't give choices to, who you can't help, like terrorists and drug addicts.'

"I almost started to laugh. Terrorists and addicts, that's who he lumps together? He wants to be a lawyer. Can you imagine?"

In some ways I thought her classmate was right. Many addicts are like terrorists, deep in seclusion, hiding out somewhere.

"The instructor claims she's an expert on addiction, whatever that means. All that I know is if I were ever a psychologist, I don't think I'd want to work in the treatment field, even though I might be good at it. Brian had a lot of counselors who were addicts, but they didn't have any education. For the most part they had licenses from one of those warehouses—three hours of school, twenty bucks, and you have a certificate.

"I still feel like an imposter every day. I feel bad for myself in school. I feel oppressed." She stopped to giggle before she went on. Laughter was a way of neutralizing terror. "Not by race or class or gender. By my own disability. I wasted college. I pissed it away completely, never mind the ten subsequent years.

"Okay. Tell me if this is bad. I bought the books for class, copied the parts I needed, and then returned them. I can't spend a hundred dollars on books. I can't believe they don't put the books on reserve. I copied them at work on Sunday." She didn't wait for me to answer. "Can I justify it? Well, I paid for the copy paper. It's not that bad a crime, is it?"

Whenever I heard Lucy use the word *crime,* I thought of her ex-boyfriend.

"Not that bad. Have you heard from Brian?"

I never go on the Internet and search for my patients or people they tell me about. I hadn't checked on Marco's supposed Xanax charge. I make no effort to find out more about patients even when so many details are available online. Whatever they choose not to tell me about is outside our relationship and I can choose to imagine it or not. I respect their secrets, accept their mysteries.

Instead, I follow up on what worries me, assuming it might worry them. Lucy was good at being casual. She told me everything as if it had bounced off her and would do the same off me. As if I were a wall and stories would carom away. But some stories adhere.

"He found out where I work. I've said it before: I'm surprised it took him so long. I was away from the store for a few days and when I got back, they told me someone had been calling but wouldn't leave a name. He left his phone number. I didn't call. A day later, I'm there when he calls again. I pick up and he says, 'This is Brian, just talk to me.' I hung up. I didn't answer the rest of the day, although I think he called three of four more times. The next day there were other people who started calling asking for me, all day long, insisting that I was the only one they could talk to, because, 'She does a really good job.' I knew Brian was having other people call.

"I think he's watching me. I have this feeling. Every call, every shadow I think is him. I don't want to go into the store anymore, but I need the money."

"You're scared." After all these months, I understood that talking was a way to distract herself from her discomfort.

"I'm freaked out. I rarely leave alone at lunch, never in the evening. The good news is that I don't think he knows anything else about me, like where I live. I've decided to get a PO box so my address is untraceable. The other good news is that my immediate reaction was not to talk to him."

"The next time he calls, why not pick up and tell him never to call you again?" We'd been over this before. She didn't look at me, but she knew when I was looking at her; if I looked for too long, it made us both uncomfortable.

"I don't know why." Her self-doubt weaved itself into our conversation whenever an opening offered itself. It was discouraging, depressing. "I should be scared of Brian when I look at it realistically. There is some reason to be scared. Men, again and again. Replicas, give or take a few years. Same MO. None of them stop.

"I'm glad he waited to contact me until I had clean time, and so long after we were involved. Now I don't have the urge to speak with him. I'm glad it didn't happen a month after starting here. I'm glad he didn't come into the store looking pathetic and sick at that point. I probably would have taken him home and we'd have had a replay. I'm afraid of relapsing again. I'm afraid of Brian. I'm afraid he'll hunt me down, we'll hop in my new car and hit my ATM machine, and it will all start up again. It's the only thing to do with him, what else would we do—go to a movie? Now there's a ridiculous thought. I couldn't ever stand his company unless I was high. He has no redeeming qualities. A tiny piece of me looked at the number he left at work and thought I could call it and start using again. That would be the only reason to call."

Even when she looked well and came in excited by the possibility of practical, worldly success—work, money to buy a new computer, good grades—she still had one foot on the other side of the gulf that separated addicts from nonaddicts. Any joy was pointless. Her fears were huge, chest crushing. What she was inclined to want (and rightly worry about wanting) was nearly always foolish, dangerous.

All addicts are thought of as impulsive, even though the schedule of opiate addiction requires forethought and discipline in acquiring drugs. Impulsivity has a purely negative connotation, but another way of describing addicts' behavior might be that they are sensation- or novelty-seeking. The initiation and continuation of drug use then, the attraction of opiates, can be thought of as a hunt for new sensations, or as a revisiting of old sensations that are taboo and illicit. Does the diminished ability to inhibit inappropriate behavior begin only after one finds pleasure (or relief) in drugs, or are certain people born with an impulsive nature? Many individuals treasure the tense excitement of the inadvisable—they lower themselves into underground caves, race snowmobiles, tame tigers. Impulsivity leads one on a quest for pleasure (Monica) or a search for a way to assuage painful feelings (Julia). But mixed into this notion of impaired self-control is an addict's enjoying the freedom to misbehave. Most addictions begin during adolescence when the world of drugs is first available and at an age when decision making is rarely deliberate. Danger is exciting and fear is far away. Personality, peers, and family are moderating influences, but some level of impairment (genetically produced?) perhaps antedates and contributes to the development of addiction. As Lucy said at her first visit, "I'll take some responsibility for things I did when I was thirteen, but I was thirteen, so how much responsibility can I take?"

Even after seeing her for nearly a year, Lucy's relentlessly secret imaginings—her impulsive craving and the need to regulate it—left me lost, confused, deluged by my inability to understand. Every day she worried about who she was and where she'd go; these concerns were never over for her. I had no great words of wisdom to offer. But then she hadn't taken Brian's call, and she hadn't called back; she had in some ways freed herself of him. Her qualms about Brian finding her were serious; she worked over and around them.

"My landlord still calls me. So I looked at a new apartment," she reported.

It was good to see her exert her will. Like Brian, her landlord needed to be avoided, not negotiated with. She was right: the men in her life were, one after the other, replicas.

"He calls, but I usually don't even listen to the message. He always has a reason for calling. I told you he's propositioned my roommates. But he doesn't call them all the time. He never had *them* in his office and closed the door and turned off the lights like he did with me after my first month there. He said, 'We could do something right here.' I started to cry. 'I didn't realize you were so sensitive,' he said."

It was there in her face, the bitter truth of who she was, another aspect of herself she couldn't grasp. In this building, to either side, there are acres of offices where patients admit to having certain thoughts they would announce nowhere else. In every room, every day there is some small dawn of understanding. Sometimes patients feel sadder and better. Sometimes sadder and worse.

"I wrote him a letter telling him I was moving out. I told him to leave me alone until I left and if he fucked with me I'd fuck with him. I wrote, 'Your behavior is inappropriate to say the least.' I'm not sure how smart he is, so I told him, 'Mess with me and it won't be hard to think of ways to mess with you.' I told him not to expect me to pay him again. The words flew off my pen. He walks around like he owns the world, like he can do anything. The world spins with people like that on it. And I meet them all."

"You certainly know a lot of them."

She knit her fingers and locked her arms behind her head. Its window sealed, the door shut, my room, when no one speaks, is a tomb.

"When I told my roommates I was moving out, they started interviewing immediately for another roommate. I was there the evening this woman came in who works at a drug treatment agency. She announced she was an addict with ten years of clean time. After she left, one of my roommates went on a rant about drug addicts and how she didn't want a junkie living there. It was vicious. 'Why can't we find another person like you?' she said to me. The irony was rich."

"You didn't reveal anything?"

"No. But I'm thinking: this is not a good thing."

"So with your family, with your roommates, you're walking around with the weight of secrets."

She looked up at me and laughed long and hard. "I don't mean to laugh. You make it sound so sinister. This is the same roommate who set me up on a date."

"You went on a date?" It was the last thing I expected to hear. She was struggling to be normal. "How was it?"

"This guy called me at work on Friday. We went out for Italian food, which was actually pretty good."

"Sounds nice."

"Being on a date was like being underwater. A weird feeling. He realized that I didn't want to be there. He kept asking, 'What's wrong? What's wrong?' It was like I was hearing him through water. After dinner, I left. 'Did I do something?' he kept asking. I understand why he was confused."

"What happened?"

"The prospect of explaining myself to another person, him or anyone else, is really not appealing. It's pointless. I remember this guy coming up to me after that meeting I went to in Hilton Head. He said to me, 'You know you're a free spirit, that's why you got into drugs.' Other people have said that to me. That it's unfortunate I got into something over my head. That I got high because I'm easygoing, happy-go-lucky, or I like the Grateful Dead or something. They think it just from the way I look, I guess.

"'What's wrong?' this guy on the date kept asking. I said, 'I have to leave.' 'Why? Talk to me. What happened? I like you,' he said. But what was I going to say? My history of men is horrendous. The only thing men are good for is to get high with."

"You sound disgusted with him."

"More with myself. I'm angry at myself. I'm a waste of human life. I've had every advantage and squandered it because I'm a lazy, hedonistic, slothful, selfish person. Incapable of having a relation-ship with anyone, mother, father, sister, people, anyone. Most days I think I'm just pathetic.

"I will never go on another date. If anything, dating makes me want to use. That and the cold weather. There's something about cuddling up with some pills in winter. Of course, there's some-thing every season, the leaves falling in autumn, steam rising off the pavement in spring, but especially summer when it's not so bad to be homeless.

"I used to have a friend who lived near the restaurant. He's dead from an overdose. I could see his house." She fell silent, which was the loudest kind of suffering.

"Did you do anything self-destructive after the date ended?" I asked apprehensively.

"Nope. I sat in my car watching the prostitutes and the drug action. I bought some gum. I went home. It was a funny way of handling things."

She sounded like a penitent. I had the sudden feeling that this was her last visit: she wasn't going to come back. The only reason she came was to get her next month's supply of pills, but she didn't want to explain herself to me anymore. I wasn't sure why I thought this, but I did. I wasn't sure what she was capable of, but it seemed like something I should know at this point about her. She was solitary; she could just walk away.

It was clear she wanted to tell me something else. At a certain point, I barely had to ask questions. I knew she was about to talk about something she hadn't talked about before, or not so in-tensely, with anyone else.

"As a kid, maybe eight years old, I had rituals. I was supersti-tious. I'd have to count the letters in every sentence to make sure they were multiples of three or my sister would die. It must have taken ninety percent of my brain capacity. I didn't tell anyone, though. I didn't realize how strange it was when I was a kid, but in the last week, when I was counting, I realized how I was trying to control my nerves."

A dazed repetition, the inability to snap out of it. She'd mentioned this during her last visit. A ritual that was curious and amazing and quieting. Like Vicodin.

"I accept anxiety that to most people would be over the top. I'm used to it." She made no plea or appeal; it was a self-pity that required nothing from me. I let her talk and didn't try to interrupt or reassure her.

"I'm pretty good at putting it out of my mind. But I always have little pictures dancing in my head. It's just a matter of how intrusive they are."

"Can you tell me about the picture that keeps coming back?" As much as I sensed she wasn't returning after this visit, I also knew her fears and anxieties must have been related to some of the stuff she'd been hesitant to talk to me about.

"There are a few, but one in particular."

For a minute, maybe two, maybe ten, she was silent. At every visit there were times when she faded, dropped back into her own thoughts, went still and distant. She squeezed her thumb between her other fingers. She put her toe on point. All of us have to believe that for those events we are reluctant to examine, history is better left untouched.

"It seems as if you're working hard not to say anything," I finally said.

"I'm not working hard at all. I'm used to not talking about it."

"Have you ever shared whatever it is you're thinking?"

"I don't think so."

In the time with me, she had never been forgetful; she denied little of what was true; she refused to answer only rarely, so when she did, I knew it was a crucial thing.

"You've carried something in your head for a long time."

"I have certain images. I really don't want to think that things that happened to me can have such a profound impact on my life twenty years later. I was eight years old. I know exactly when it was. I remember what was on TV that night, the show and who was on it. I thought it was half a dream, but I went online and found the show and when it aired. May 15, 1985, a Saturday night."

She started slowly, remembering as she spoke, often pausing to look into space, to relive it. She sometimes paused to search for the right word.

"My father was not at home. He was out of town. My mother was asleep. Dana was in a bassinet near my mother's bed. I was sleeping in the next room. I heard Dana crying. I went in to her room and picked her up and put her into the bed next to my mother and I slid in next to her. She was between me and my mother. I quieted her for a while. Then I went to sleep. My mother said she never even knew we got into bed with her. In the morning, Dana didn't move. My mother couldn't wake Dana up. She lifted her in her blanket and Dana didn't make a sound. I remember my mother started screaming. She was screaming at me and at Dana.

"For years I thought: if only I hadn't fallen asleep. If only I had paid better attention. Some days I wondered: if I hadn't been lying so close to her; on other days, if I had only been nearer."

Sometimes in my office, the sound of disaster is silence, not a crash. I needed to clear my throat, but the room was too quiet. Neither of us moved. Our breathing had stopped. There were no words. As with every patient, when I started to ask Lucy questions, I understood that I might hear things I wished I hadn't. But even when she was finished, I never guessed the extent this would be the case.

I felt nauseated. It was unbearable to think of Lucy as a little girl that day.

Her baby sister had disappeared, she was simply gone, gone from the earth without a trace. As if the baby had disappeared in a dream.

As an eight-year-old, some part of Lucy must have believed her sister would come back. Eight-year-olds are unsure of death, cannot know its permanence. Would she always be dead? Would she see her again? Her sister would walk in one day, and Lucy would be waiting. Her sister would call or come in a door. If only Lucy could find just the right word or signal or combination of numbers. She must have allowed the possibility that her sister would return. Maybe she still did.

But at the same time, Lucy knew she would never touch her, play with her or see her face, or hear her voice or feel her breath. Life had been split in two—when her baby sister was alive and when she wasn't.

The guilt: Had she killed her sister? Who would ever forgive her? She was the only witness; she must have been the cause. I wanted to shout, *There was nothing that could have been done—everyone knew that.* But no one could convince her, had ever convinced her, that it wasn't her fault. I saw her across the room, sitting mute with the impossibility of knowing what had really happened.

There was no way to stop the guilt except to forget it. For twenty years she had been engaged in the act of forgetting. One night when she was thirteen and found her parents' liquor, she discovered a way to blot out the sickening future. Later, Vicodin helped obliterate memory. It helped counteract the wrongness and the loss. With Vicodin, the numbness reinforced a sense of being alone, where no one could bother her. With Vicodin, time closed over her; she stopped glimpsing back. It was a cloak to hide from the world. Or maybe a way of killing herself so she could see her sister again.

But the terror remained. Twin terrors: Was I the cause of my sister's death? Will I die in some horrible silent way, too? As a girl she had been afraid of many things, she'd told me. Loud noises, heights, driving behind garbage trucks, food that could get caught in her throat, very fat people, bicycle gears. She was still afraid: of men, homelessness, poverty. What could be more impoverished than a baby's empty bassinet? She'd told me she had no maternal instincts. Of course not. And not because she had been sexually or physically abused as a child like so many of my patients. She had suffered terribly in another way. There was a piece of her missing; she was unbalanced. Her life was punitive. She tested all the dangers out there with Vicodin as consolation. It required a greater and different courage to move past the danger. Would there ever be a time without terror?

I had been convinced she had been abused. Where did I get the idea? Had she ever implied it? Her father's temper? His failure to ever make her feel safe? Really, what did I know about her? I had only been right in understanding that her eyes on my door had a deeper meaning than opiate dependence alone might account for.

My mother's younger brother died of polio when he was five years old and she was ten. When he got sick, she had been sent away to live with an aunt and uncle on a farm a hundred miles from the city so as not to become infected herself. She never saw her curly-haired brother alive again. Rather than try to forget, she kept his picture in her room her entire life. Her memory of him was a journey back to places they had been together. This was her consolation even during her years with dementia.

Was there any consolation I could offer Lucy? Should I have told her about my mother, who had her own images and ghostly memories and terrors?

I realized that Lucy had never said my name, first or last.

Would it have mattered to her that my uncle had died when he was five years old?

"I used to ask my mother to bring me to doctors because I had strange pains," she said quietly. "I probably said something vague to them, and they didn't know what to do for me. I tried to talk to her, but she didn't listen. But I think my mother knew how upset I was. Once, as a teenager, we had a fight in the car and I basically told her and my father that I was a bad person. I was horrifying and would never be forgiven. My father didn't pick up on it, but she did. I know she did. Picked up on it in her usual way and didn't say anything. Years later she once said to me, 'Those things that happened to you are not your fault.'"

Not every conversation with a patient ranged so far. Most patients head straight for what hurts or is physically noticeable and never budge from the newly offending symptoms. Even if I start with, "Why don't you tell me what I should know about you to best care for you," most patients do not want to go very deeply into what has been wonderful for them in life, or intolerable. But some do. Some offer a past no one knew about until they came to my office.

Lucy must have felt, still felt, she had done something horrendous, more than careless. What kind of person would let her baby sister die? A person who was pathetic, a failure. She'd never get over it.

But was that true? I'd met many patients over the years who had suffered terribly and had not become addicts; who somehow mastered adversity, and even transformed their difficulties into productive lives; who used their own important and traumatic events as resources, as a way to move into life; who had not been frozen in the awful past but had broken apart the icy conspiracy of circumstance.

Why had she been unable to become a "normie" like her sister, who also grew up in a house where a baby had died? Was Lucy born with a neurological system so reactive to painful memories it required constant numbing, whereas those who escaped addiction were wired to find other ways to handle aversive thoughts? Had her relationship with her parents—who must have retreated into grief at one daughter's death and minimized the surviving daughters' problems—contributed to Lucy seeking an alternate reality?

Lucy's guilt was so strong she had to do something self-destructive. She once told me she didn't care if her body rotted. She told me she wasn't sure she could put the effort into taking care of herself. "If I cared about myself," she said, "I wouldn't have done all these things to myself."

CHAPTER 10

Friday, April 9

This year I turned away more than one opiate addict seeking buprenorphine. This morning, during my first patient visit, I saw the light on my phone begin blinking as a phone call came in silently. It was a message, a threat really, from a fifty-year-old woman whom I'd seen last week and refused entry into my program because she was taking high doses of a tranquilizer in addition to high doses of Vicodin. She was receiving both from a doctor in another part of the state whom she told me she would continue to see despite my suggestion that he might not be doing her a service. When I listened to this message, I heard her say, "I've got a big complaint about you. You better take that white jacket off because you're not a professional. You're not going to decide my fate. You're an idiot and I need to talk to you. My number is 987–2321 and my name is Carol. Call me before I get you and fucking strangle you."

Of course, I wasn't going to call back, but the whole thing put me in a strange state and made me a little shaky after I put down the receiver. She was so full of rage and at the same time she was begging for her life.

At home, in middle age, I often feel that I am waiting for something to happen. I have no interest in peace of mind; agitation is fine with me. I am ready for action, for change and improvement, for seeing things differently. In the office, with patients, I look for responses to the therapy I offer. I watch for the transformations I expect—the swelling disappeared, the inflamed skin's redness abated. How do I keep track of all that was changing? I make lists. I have a list of patient diagnoses or symptoms in the chart that I copy from one written note to the next as the sleep apnea, the arthritis of the left knee, the pedal edema, and the erectile difficulty improve or worsen, never staying the same from one visit to the next.

For another year I had refused to decorate like my colleagues have. Laura had colorful wall hangings and wooden statues from Malawi. My colleague Max, after an extended trip to Fiji, now had dried anemones and starfish and sponges on his tabletops; his office looks like a beach town in the off-season. My room with its sameness and simplicity offers a sense of perpetual return to patients, and to me.

I opened Lucy Fields's chart on my desk in preparation for her next visit. What did she know about me after all this time? Could she know, after a year of seeing me wear a tie, that I despised them? Did she know I'd ironed my blue shirt this morning, on the floor of my room, pressing it on a blanket? Did she realize I'd held out for longer than I thought possible against my sons' plea for a flat-screen TV? Was she aware I had refinished the desk from my grandfather's medical office and now worked on it at home in the evenings? To Lucy, I was a man of industry with hunched shoulders, alone in the small geography of his office.

What did I know about her? I had an itemized list, under the heading "Drug Use," of the parts of her life that needed care and improvement: Fear, Men, Sex, Parents, Craving, Money, School. Looking at the list, I was struck by how well she had begun to reassemble her entire existence piece by piece.

"For some reason I still believe that I could have a meaningful life." I remembered how strangely worry free she had seemed during her first visit. Smooth-browed. In retrospect, it was probably just the Vicodin. The sinister, violent, and dangerous lurked near Lucy, but for a moment that morning, they were poised and hidden. I had looked for the damage. She was lucky she had never ended up bloodied, or worse. She was also confident she could get through another day in her foul utopia if things didn't work out with me. She didn't want me to see her addiction as her fault. She agreed right off that she had brought it on herself, but she was clearly bothered by the word *fault*. Her problem was the result of her behavior, but she hadn't asked for the problem as a young teenager, she'd told me.

The question that first day was whether she'd look at me. The question was not whether she'd speak. If she didn't speak, I'd wait. At the time I didn't understand that when she stared at my door, she was staring into memory. She was lost in time. But during her last few visits, I'd felt that a decade of masochism was ending. She had accepted the grotesque and grim, every failure and inequity, even if she still didn't believe that they were forgivable.

The last visit had been a turning point. She had trusted me

with something that was not small. Trust is a moral choice, like bravery, and I was honored. I don't know anyone who particularly likes what they see in the mirror, but I remembered the way Lucy always ducked when she passed the mirror en route to her chair. Yet when we'd last seen each other, she had looked into herself and offered me her story, not as a way to fix herself, but perhaps as a way of not being alone any longer with a part of her life that couldn't be solved or fled.

When I tell friends about my addicted patients, they want to know: How did this catastrophe arise? But the more patients I've seen, the more I've come to understand that biography should never be taken for granted, that it is nearly always uninformed to believe that one can draw a straight line from childhood trauma to grown-up behavior. The jumble of personality, support, accomplishment, and love; the means to self-organize, self-regulate, and self-console; the storm of human details was too dense and intricate to explain why one person at thirty has a sense of purpose while another has had just about enough of life. Broken childhoods might lead to adulthoods that are uneasy or self-respecting; poetic, dreary, or metaphysical; or addicted. In my office, when patients offer painful personal history it is sometimes as proof of survival and sometimes in the hope that I will see them more clearly. It is also sometimes a declaration of independence from the brutalities of the past.

Lucy came in wearing black sandals, jeans, and a crimson T-shirt. Her eyes were a light-absorbing color, made even darker by a touch of mascara. Her skin was darker as well. She had a pretty silver necklace with an irregular white stone pendant. She wore nail polish. She sat sideways on her chair and put her Alice Munro paperback on the floor beside her next to the black knit purse, its drawstring pulled tight. She held on to her coffee in its silver thermos.

"Three weeks ago, before I went to South Carolina, they gave me high school students to work with at the store. Two kids from a city-sponsored program for disadvantaged youth who are actually paid to work at the store on Saturdays from nine to three. They had to be better than I was at that age, less problematic, I thought. I was drinking or using drugs every day when I was fifteen. These two complained nonstop—why do we have to do this, why do we have to do that? It wasn't just me, everyone who came in contact with them got frustrated with their whining.

"So listen to this," she said, giggling. "Last Saturday they came back from lunch high. I told them, 'Get out of here. You guys know that when you get high something happens, there are consequences.' I was leaning toward firing at least one of them, anyway, they were so unpleasant as a pair. But I had to fire them both for getting high. It's kind of funny, don't you think? Now the district manager likes me because of my uncanny ability to sniff out drug use."

She laughed a big belly laugh. "They weren't even smart enough to deny it. If they had any brains they would have. What was their defense? 'Everybody does it. Other kids get high.' 'It's not up to me,' I told them. Marie was considering suspending them for a week, but there was a big powwow and the district manager said, 'Are you joking? No way.' Anyway, my job on Saturdays just got much easier."

"So they must *really* appreciate you at work."

"Not Marie. Who knows what sets her off? I can tell when I walk in the door if she's going to be abusive that day. I think I've become too functional for her. She likes people who are needy and dependent and have mind-boggling problems. That's the way she saw me when I first got there, afraid of being homeless, willing to take just about anything. I don't feel I'm like that anymore.

"I want you to know that the idea that anything, let alone this pill I've been taking, can make me better leaves me in disbelief."

"It seems to me you're better than when you first came in."

"I'm biding time until the next disaster." She smiled. "I went tanning last night. I stood in a box. Twelve minutes, the maximum allowed by law. I wanted to keep the tan I got in South Carolina."

"That's the third time in a year you've been to see your parents by my count," I pointed out. Some days she arrived looking as if she had other things she needed to do, some days she sat heavily, as if she had no place to go. Today she seemed relaxed, her face loosened. She worked her hands, rubbing them as if they were cold.

"This time they were on some weird macrobiotic diet. My mother's been on a diet since she was twelve years old, but this one is far-fetched even for her—brown rice and seaweed. She has my father on it. They made me eat it, too.

"She told me I'm better with no lunatic boyfriends around. She's always blamed my life on my boyfriends. I was not in the mood to enlighten her or argue with her. I think the vinegar's gone to her head."

She giggled. I thought: the mother had the nerve to pity the daughter while all the while she was being pitied.

"Did I tell you that my sister is pregnant? She called me. She left messages for me at work. I didn't call her for a few days. I figured something was wrong that she needed to tell me and I didn't want to hear it.

" 'You're going to be an aunt,' she said, when I finally called her back from Hilton Head. 'I'm due in October.' 'Congratulations,' I said. 'You excited?' she asked me.

"Actually I think I am, more than I thought I'd be. I wasn't totally surprised, although they did go to work on the baby creation pretty fast. I talked to her husband at the wedding and he told me that he wanted kids.

"My sister told my mother first and wasn't even going to call me, but my mother actually confronted her about the way she's treated me since the wedding. You know what my sister told her? She said, 'Lucy ignored me when we were growing up. She wasn't the sister I needed.'

"My sister sent me an e-mail asking me to apologize for not being a good sister. So I did. Of course, I'm not the sole cause of our relationship going wrong at this point. But I e-mailed her back an apology in order to keep some semblance of a relationship. I also told her why it happened, that I suffer from at least one mental illness, namely addiction. You know what she responded? 'I know you have issues.'"

I tried to think of them as children. As a teenager, her sister probably wanted Lucy to teach her to put on makeup, talk about boys, treat her with special affection, speak about the death of their younger sister, and Lucy probably wasn't capable of any of it.

"I know this baby will be the test of our relationship. I have no interest in him or her. I don't really like children. I don't find them cute or adorable. But I know when he or she is born I will send a gift, just like I did for their wedding so they don't think that I'm a destitute loser."

"Do you think that will help?"

"It may. Expensive gifts matter in her world. They're status symbols."

"I give you a lot of credit for making these efforts with your family," I said.

"I won't have a relationship with them ever if I don't. People need family, right? Not that I ever expect my sister to help me, and I'll never ask her for anything. She would let me die in a shelter and not help me."

"But you reached out. Of course your attention to her and her new baby may not immediately make up for all the resentment she expressed in her e-mail."

"I'm really not sure I did anything so bad to her. She asked me to apologize for something that at this point is the result of a serious problem. You shouldn't ask your sister to apologize for mental illness. But it's always been entirely my fault. Every family dysfunction is blamed on me.

"In class, they gave us this case of a girl in the projects, sixteen years old, who'd go on crack binges. To keep her off drugs, her parents chained her to the radiator in their apartment with the tacit consent of the neighbors. They brought her food; she watched cable TV all day. I didn't know who I thought was right. Do I think the parents should go to prison for violating her rights? No. Do I condone what they did to her? No. I understand both sides, but it made me angry about why my parents didn't do more for me. They should have helped me more. Why didn't they? I used to think they were stingy, or afraid, or were unwilling to believe the worst.

"I guess we're still in collusion that my situation is not as bad as it looks. That's what they want to think and what I want them to think. They think I've been clean for five years, not one. I've got to keep some secrets, don't I?" she said, self-knowingly.

After a moment, she announced, "I bought a car."

"What kind?"

"A Kia."

I looked out the window, as if it were parked just below. Through the rectangular frame of glass, the nearby building seemed almost magnified; I saw every angle of the Children's

Hospital clearly. I stared for a while as if I could hear some of the action on the street. "What color?"

"Red. I thought it was safe being a thousand miles away from my parents, but for months my mother's been working on me to get a car. Every time she calls, she asks, 'You have to take three buses to school? What if it rains? What if you have to come home at night?'"

I agreed with her mother. My son had recently started taking the bus across town from school in the afternoon. He had to connect to a second line at the downtown plaza where half the commuters were addicts, and the other half were plainclothes police. After twenty years living in this state, I'd never ridden a bus. I couldn't imagine life without a car.

"God forbid someone in her family doesn't drive a car, or drives an old car," Lucy continued. "It's inexpensive and it actually drives pretty well and it's not as small inside as I thought. But now I'm saddled with a new car I'm not sure I even want. I still feel like it isn't mine. I still expect to look out my window and see the repo man seizing it."

"He wouldn't do that."

"He would if my father weren't putting in $200 a month toward the payment. They've backed off from their fiscal austerity line. At a certain point they thought I was old enough to take care of myself, I wasn't their responsibility. Their age cutoff was somewhere around twenty-two. At that point they thought their duty expired. That would have been fine under normal conditions. It's not bad to teach your children to support themselves. But this wasn't normal circumstances."

"So you like your new Kia." I wanted to hear her say she adored it. I kept trying to steer her toward an admission of pleasure. Over the last months it had become clear that she kept herself from thinking or feeling certain things. My job, it seemed, was to make her more self-conscious, to make her alert to the small satisfactions that might someday take the place of Vicodin. I had been trying from day one to reset her habitual negativity. I wanted her automatic answers (and behaviors) to become less automatic.

"It makes it easier to get around, that's for sure. Since I got back from South Carolina, I've found myself driving around the old neighborhoods nearly every day, the neighborhoods where I used to go with Brian. But this week I was thinking about why I was driving there when I'm not really interested in using. Am I really trying to find drugs? No, or I *would* find them. I started to think: What if I'm saying good-bye? It's starting to sink in that I might never use again. That never using again might be possible. What is the feeling? Melancholy? I remember the good and the bad. I'm feeling things now I should have been feeling then, but wasn't.

"I was driving yesterday and when I got to a turn we used to make onto Academy Avenue, I didn't take it. I realized that if I give myself long enough to think about using, I don't use. That's the clearheadedness I have now. When I was a girl, my father used to tell me, 'Before you do anything, think it out to the conclusion. Here's what will happen.' But I wasn't capable of that when I was taking Vicodin every day. When you are in the routine of using, you don't do much thinking. Thinking doesn't mean anything. Now, I don't have to take it to the conclusion. I know what the conclusion will be."

Lucy had always wanted to explain her behavior to me; most addicts do, even if it involves their greatest guilt, even if it results in self-denunciation. They want to make themselves *less* unacceptable. With Lucy, I had tried to take a posture of steadfast forgiveness. It wasn't hard, my heart went out to her. In the past months, my office had become a place where regret was stilled, anxiety muted, memory made transparent; and what existed was mournful awareness.

For months now, I had had an image of Lucy as a functional adult. But there was another way I had to think of her. As someone who would always struggle with the humiliation of fifteen years of using Vicodin and the worry of being crazy. As someone who would never lead the life she could have led. She imagined a harsher fate perhaps—an early death. But it hadn't happened and now she had the trappings of a normal life: she was living in a small apartment, working, going to school. She would progress. She would forever wrangle with her mother, father, and sister over the meaning of what had gone before. Her reentry into conventionality would be slow and difficult.

Over the years I had become resigned to seeing people who, for the moment, were not quite getting what they wanted out of life.

Lucy was sitting on her chair like a catcher behind home plate, but facing me for a change as I pitched more questions on this close-to-a-year-anniversary visit. We talked about her father who was miserable about South Carolina's newest gun laws, and more about her mother's belief in prolonged life through seaweed. We talked about unpaid student loans and the cost of a cable TV package she wanted. We talked again about her fear of homelessness and how she'd had to pay the bank for years of overdrawn and bounced check fees in order to open an account.

Was Vicodin a self-protective response to her family and personal history? I wondered again: If Lucy had come to her first visit complaining of a pain with no clear, explicable cause, and had told me she'd tried a Vicodin and found it helped some with this unnameable pain, but helped even more with mood and day-to-day feeling, if she had told me she had started it as an antidepressant but was now using ten Vicodin a day and her body had gotten used to it, that is, became dependent on it, would I have thought as badly of her as I did of Dan of the tapping feet who came in that same week and wouldn't admit to a Percocet problem but wanted a prescription? If I had given her Vicodin and she had been one of the millions of Americans with undiagnosable pain who did *not* misuse it—showing up once a month for a supply and using exactly the number she was given—that is, if she wasn't abusing Vicodin, would that have been so bad? Would it have been different from her using buprenorphine?

But I knew certain questions would have always gnawed at me—did she really need an opiate at all? Was there another, nonaddictive medicine or therapy that would help with her mood, and which in turn would ameliorate her pain? What if this dependence had started in the midst of a pain that was going to go away on its own? What if her pain, while chronic, did not really limit her? How close was Lucy to being any of these hypothetical persons? Was the way she responded to opiates an affliction or a human variant? Had I been programmed by my training and my culture to believe the chronic use of Vicodin was *always* asking for trouble, or was I willing to accept that we all did things that were a little unsatisfactory so that in some way we could be happier? Maybe certain people find their way to the best therapy for themselves, even if that therapy isn't socially sanctioned.

Why did Lucy trade Vicodin for buprenorphine a year ago? The standard answer everyone wanted to hear—drugs are ruining my life—was the answer opiate-dependent patients gave. But it was only half the answer, because drugs had been ruining their lives for months or years (although in some ways drugs also made life manageable) by the time they tried to quit. I needed to hear something beyond this, a broader motive that explained the timing of a first visit to my office. What it often came down to was an unacceptable level of self-hatred, grief cascading like a waterfall, which in Lucy's case she experienced as fatigue: I'm tired.

Even when she was using, the first day she came to see me, she looked ordinary. Nearly every addict does, despite how they are depicted in movies. Only after Lucy told her story did it become clear that she had aberrant needs that had crippled her for a decade. Anyone could look at her—lanky and long-haired, her eyes down as she walked quickly past—and think they knew the life she'd been living. But they didn't. If there is anything doctoring teaches, it is that routine human business is unfathomable.

"It sounded as if things were pretty good with your parents this visit."

"They told me they were proud of me. But it's sad because I'll probably end up disappointing them." She had something to celebrate and yet it sounded as if she'd been granted another stay of execution, her case still under appeal.

"My thirtieth birthday is coming up in a few days," she said. "I don't think of myself as thirty. More like fifteen."

Fifteen years old—I knew it well from my younger son. The age of mocking and scorn, of resenting the world of rules and regulations. The age of impatience, filled with a desire to know and feel everything all the time. At fifteen, my son wanted to be thirty with a driver's license, a car, and cash in his pocket. But who would do his laundry or bring him soup when he was sick? Lucy was already an addict at fifteen—hidden, unappreciated.

At fifteen, drugs must have given her a sense of identity, a transgressive glamour and pride from hanging out with older guys. At fifteen, whatever she imagined as a career was far off. Accomplishment wasn't on her mind, just cough syrup and hallucinogens. As she grew older, more experience with drugs and men must have made her feel street smart; with Mark and then Brian she took on an outlaw aspect. Then more years of inertia. Now she was thirty.

"I don't think of myself as thirty. More like fifteen." Did she mean it was painful to define herself again? Did she mean she no longer felt distinctive and had to face the prosaic world like everyone else?

I thought: at her age, at thirty, I was married and had a child.

"My mother used to say I wasn't comfortable in my own skin. She's right. The only thing I was ever good at was being a drug addict. That was the only thing I've done successfully."

She sounded nostalgic. As if the years living with Brian, locked indoors and using thirty Vicodin a day recalled a simpler time. This kind of distortion hid a fear of the future, a yearning for order and safety, qualities that hadn't graced her life since she was seven years old.

"It didn't sound so successful to me."

"If success means taking it as far as you can without dropping dead, I was pretty successful," she said with her typical black humor.

I wasn't going to let her sink again.

She was thin and looked fragile, but I knew she was tough. She had given up drugs, and what was left was anguish. She hadn't spread herself over the chair, but was keeping herself within its limits. She was facing me.

"You've had a good number of successes this year," I said. "But I'm not surprised it's hard for you. This is all good. Can you remember what you were like a year ago?"

"I can. It feels like there's a thin line between that life and this one. Most days it feels like that was a totally different person, that

I'm talking about another person, which is a scary feeling. Brian yelling and pushing; that was my day-to-day life. One horrible thing after another and it went on and on. It's hard thinking about that person who cared so little about herself. I'm not blaming myself for other people's behavior, but that I put myself there and couldn't get out and that I repeated the pattern for ten years is frightening. I'm not even sure what stopped it. The pinnacle was the day I came here. There was nothing particularly bad that day, but for some reason I felt the accumulated size and weight of it and it kind of hit me."

Her thirtieth birthday was this week and I thought we should celebrate. With some patients there is always a sense of some faint discomfort: we aren't able to talk; we aren't a good match. But Lucy Fields and I got along. I'd listened to her speak about her life in a struggling, moving way and if you asked why there was an affinity, what she said or did that stirred a warm feeling in me, I still couldn't have said exactly. Listening to her had taught me what people will ignore or forget. Listening had taught me the mechanisms people employ to tuck away the intolerable, the incongruous, the disruptive. I listened as if listening would save her. I listened as if it would strip away her anger and self-reproach. I had the luxury of listening because she didn't need to be interrogated—she did that to herself.

"At my first visit, when you said I had to come back in five days, I couldn't believe it. You basically said I should use for five more days before you would medicate me."

"But you came back."

"I really did want something to change. I started listening to a little thing in my head that said: there's a chance you can live. At other times in my life I'd felt I really wanted to change, but I guess that feeling didn't last. To come back from a lifelong problem is next to impossible. I don't know where my determination came from. Sometimes I think—and I'm not religious—that something stepped in, some force, and said, 'You have to do something with your life.' I've certainly had more determination this time than ever before."

I've seen Lucy for three years now. She talks easily when she comes into my office every month. She no longer seems wary. She is halfway through graduate school.

Why does a doctor find his interest in one place and not another? So much of medical practice depends on one's ability to demand and receive a change in a patient's behavior. Addicts are my greatest challenge. If I present advice on health and longevity as a series of "You shoulds," addicts see life as a series of "Why should I's?" This challenge is messy and time-consuming and I love every minute of it. On any given day when I'm talking with Lucy, Julia, Marco, Monica, and Joe, I don't know if it's morning or afternoon. The hours pass. I've been bored only once or twice in all these years.

Julia still tries to sell herself as a good patient. She has stayed on buprenorphine far longer than she thought she would, and she has remained Vicodin free. She holds in a lot of what she might tell me, surprised she has told me as much as she has. "I never thought a doctor would ask me so many questions," she said recently. But it's taken her months to admit she'd begun to buy Xanax on the street for those days when she felt more stress than she could handle. Too often with me she retreats into shame.

Chef Marco has never returned. Monica lost control of her weekend heroin use, lost her job a year ago, moved into a residential treatment program for three months, stopped all opiate use, and sees me twice a year for asthma care. Joe, my handyman, weaned off buprenorphine; the only medication I give him now is for hypertension.

I do not accept that addiction is like quicksand where the more one struggles, the deeper one sinks. But the first call for help is always a dismaying, humiliating prospect. To work with addicts is to enter the profession of possibility; holding off the submersion into relapse has to be an improvisation. There is a risk of false dreams and false confidence. The silence of my office helps to accommodate the many patients who deteriorate into apprehension and rage. I barely move. I absorb their losses and wishes. A simple nod signals competence. I have failures and successes.

At every visit, I am moved by how Lucy had been brought so low, and how much she has regained. I look around my office as she does; it remains unadorned, sensible, counter and exam table and desk too close to one another. I stare out the window. The trees are nearly back to the way they were when this smart young woman first arrived. The triple-decker owners have held out another year, refusing to sell to the hospital, which relentlessly seeks property to expand its parking lots. The two skimpy front yards have newly painted fences. One has a birdbath with a pale blue bowl.

Acknowledgments

I'm grateful to all the patients who let me into their lives. Through each, I come to know the world a little more.

I am fortunate to be edited by Henry Ferris, who insists on precision. He worked at least as hard as I did on every sentence in this book.

Betsy Lerner has taught me to first trust my writing instincts and later to trust hers. Her aim is true and her friendship dear.

Each evening, Hester, Toby, and Alex ask about my day and hear these stories first. Delighting them remains my greatest delight.